D0282983

Healthy Heart Handbook

How to prevent and reverse
heart disease, lower your risk of
heart attack and cancer, reduce stress
and lose weight without hunger

Dr. Neal Pinckney

Health Communications, Inc.
Deerfield Beach, Florida

An earlier version of this work was previously issued in a limited prepublication edition by the Healing Heart Foundation.

This book is not intended to be a substitute for medical advice. Before you start any lifestyle change in diet or exercise, it is strongly recommended that you consult with a physician/health professional who can evaluate your individual physical condition and advise you about any special considerations.

Position of the American Dietetic Association: Vegetarian Diets was published in the Journal of the American Dietetic Association, November 1993, Volume 93, Number 11. Reprinted by permission. The American Dietetic Association, 216 West Jackson Boulevard, Chicago, IL 60606-6995.

Library of Congress Cataloging-in-Publication Data

Pinckney, Neal.
  Healthy heart handbook : how to prevent and reverse heart disease, lower your risk of heart attack and cancer, reduce stress, lose weight without hunger / Neal Pinckney.
    p.   cm.
  "An earlier version of this work was previously published in a limited prepublication edition by the Healing Heart Foundation"—t.p. verso.
  Includes bibliographical references and index.
  ISBN 1-55874-384-7 (trade paper)
  1. Coronary heart disease—Prevention. 2. Coronary heart disease—Nutritional aspects. 3. Low-fat diet—Recipes. I. Title.
  RC685.C6P56 1996
  616.1'2305—dc20   96-6086
                                                                    CIP

©1994, 1996 Neal Pinckney
ISBN 1-55874-384-7

Publisher: Health Communications, Inc.
          3201 S.W. 15th Street
          Deerfield Beach, Florida 33442-8190

Cover design by Lawna Patterson Oldfield
Cover art illustration by TechPool Studios
Technical illustrations by Neal Pinckney

*To the loving memory of my father,
Leo Allen Pinckney (1902-1961),
who died of a heart attack at 59,
and who might be alive today
had this information
been available*

*For Andrew Allen,
Jennifer Elizabeth and
Matthew Ian*

Contents

Part One: Healthy Heart Primer

Part Two: A Healthy Heart Cookbook
66 Very Low-Fat Vegetarian Dishes

Basics

Snacks

Treats

Illustrations

Figures

Charts

Tables

Acknowledgments

The information shared here comes from many different sources. Dean Ornish, M.D., showed that heart disease is reversible and preventable; his research and writing is at the heart of this book. John McDougall, M.D., revealed the role of nutrition in many diseases, and Ruth Heidrich's example provided challenge and inspiration. More than 450 participants in my *Healing Heart* support groups shared their experiences, reactions and encouragement. This book is their story as much as mine.

Hundreds of participants from many mailing lists and Usenet newsgroups on the Internet computer network have contributed information used in this book. An especially treasured resource continues to be Michelle Dick's *Fat Free* list.

There are many people who assisted in making this book possible, too many to name in this limited space. I am indebted to three friends who edited the manuscript. William Harris, M.D., advised on medical and nutritional points. Walter McKibben, a world-class athlete for over 45 years, scrutinized it and made dozens of helpful suggestions, and Raymond Corsini, Ph.D., author and editor of some 40 books, spent many hours suggesting ways to make it more readable. Any remaining errors are solely my own responsibility.

Preface

This book has a simple objective: to save your life.

Health experts say about 70 percent of deaths from heart attacks can be prevented with lifestyle changes. But just prolonging life isn't enough. The quality of those added years is equally important. To live life to the fullest, a person has to feel good, be free from pains and physical limitations, and look forward eagerly to tomorrow. How to make this happen is what this book is all about.

Every 25 seconds, someone in America has a heart attack. And every 45 seconds, a person dies of heart disease, the number one killer of both men and women in the United States. People are dying from a lifetime of making poor choices based on *not* knowing what was good or bad for their body.

But this book is not about dying; it is about *living*. About getting back control of your health, feeling your best, having more energy, and reversing heart disease and lowering the risk of a heart attack. This means learning better choices about what goes into the body, how it is used and abused, and how factors outside the body affect the inside of it. This knowledge is not new, nor is it a well-kept secret. It is amazingly close to common sense (which doesn't seem to be as common as it used to be).

According to the U. S. Centers for Disease Control, four major factors affect your health:

CHART P.1. MAJOR FACTORS AFFECTING HEALTH

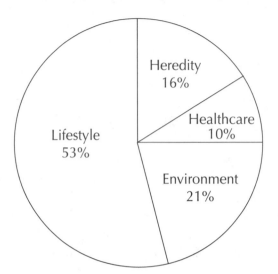

The one thing we have the ability to control by ourselves, our lifestyle, has more to do with our health than the other three factors combined.

At first I thought I learned about heart disease the hard way. When my physician told me I had triple-vessel coronary artery disease, fear and anxiety overwhelmed me. I thought I had been given a death sentence. Now I realize that my education came the easy way, compared with the hundreds of thousands who learned about heart disease from their own angioplasty or open-heart surgery. My education came painlessly, compared with those who learned about heart disease by suffering heart attacks, strokes or frantic emergency trips to the hospital.

I learned many things following my diagnosis of severe coronary artery disease. Much of it conflicted with what I read in the popular press and what I was told by some medical advisors. I learned that we can control our own present and future health much more than we had ever been led to believe. I learned how we can better take care of our bodies, properly maintaining them, protecting them from damaging elements, giving our bodies the right fuel and avoiding abusing them. Some of us take better care of our cars than we do our bodies.

The information I sought is available, but it's not always easy to find. Having a private practice and teaching at a university for nearly 30 years gave me the tools to find the information I needed and to analyze it. Being retired allowed me the time to put it all together, and being told I had a limited time to live gave me the incentive to analyze it as soon as I could.

What is known about heart disease is the cumulative work of countless dedicated physicians, research scientists and a host of other professionals. The information in this book is from clinical experiments, the experience of private practice and the writings of many experts, pioneers of a view that we can be responsible for our own health. The research and writings of Dean Ornish, M.D., stand out among all others. The diet plans of John McDougall, M.D., have allowed many to reverse illnesses and stop taking powerful drugs. When these pioneers first published their advice about alternate ways of reversing heart disease and preventing many health problems, they went "against the grain" of mainstream medical thinking. Since they first paved the way, America has become more health- and nutrition-conscious. Numerous studies have substantiated their basic ideas. Still, many medical practitioners and dieticians appear to be unaware of these findings. Worse, some choose to ignore what is likely to become a future direction for all medicine and especially for reversing heart disease, preferring to stay rooted in past beliefs.

This book may offer information that is different from what your doctor has told you. There are many reasons for this, and it does not necessarily mean that your doctor is wrong. Every person has a unique medical and physical situation. There may be reasons, some you are not aware of, that shape the advice your physician gives you. You should be able to ask your doctor questions, getting explanations for any course of treatment and medications prescribed. If you don't get answers that make sense to you, you cannot take control over your own body and life. If your physician does not give you understandable answers, find a physician willing to give them to you. When you have a physician who communicates (someone who *listens* to you as well as explains things), follow the advice you're given. Do not alter medications or dosages without first discussing any changes with your doctor. Talk over any major lifestyle changes you plan to make, including the ones recommended here. Know what your cholesterol and triglyceride levels are. Ask for the results of important tests you've taken and write the numbers down to keep in a permanent record. Take responsibility for knowing more about your body and the condition it's in.

There are a number of things you can do to reduce the risk of a heart attack and reverse heart disease. Those you can do on your own are given the most attention here. Other methods that can also be helpful in the reversal process are explained briefly, due to the limits of this book. To explain and demonstrate meditation and yoga, for example, would take another book far larger than this one.

Many of the participants in *Healing Heart* support groups asked me to put this information in a book so they could share it with family and friends. This book is the result of that effort, and it also includes the cumulative wisdom, advice and experiences of many of the participants of these support groups.

I've tried to make this book readable. It's important that every medical or nutritional statement be based on material that is from recognized peer review journals and other standard reference sources. To satisfy the scientists, there should be a footnote or other link to the reference source used, but when this was done, it looked more like a medical textbook than the guidebook it strives to be. As a compromise, all sources are listed in the bibliography.

This book is for you—to help you prevent heart attacks and surgery and to reduce your dependence on powerful medicines. It also strives to put you back in control and to make the quality of your life as good as it can be. Amazingly, you can do this and still spend less money on food, medications and treatment than you may be expending now.

When measures of protein, carbohydrates and fat are given in this book, it is usually in their percentage of total calories. Water and other substances not metabolized for energy may be a large part of what we eat or drink, sometimes close to all of it.

Label claims can be very misleading. Some claim foods are a certain percent fat-free, but that is usually the percentage of total weight. A label may claim that lunch meat is 97 percent fat free, but actually over half its calories may come from fat. To show how that can happen, let me ask you if you'd be willing to swallow two tablespoons of lard right now. Most people would refuse this offer. But if I mixed those two tablespoons of lard in a quart of warm water, added a little artificial sweetener, flavor and color and labeled it "97 percent fat-free" (that would be correct for total weight), and put on an attractive label calling it a quick energy drink, you might be tempted. Since the water doesn't count as a nutritional source, 100 percent of the 240 calories in that drink would come from fat.

PART ONE

Healthy Heart
Primer

1

How It All Began

Denial is not a river in Egypt.

I frequently saw my father, who died of a heart attack at 59, doubled over with pain. He called it "indigestion." Years later, when I was shoveling dirt in my yard and a tightness across my chest kept me from continuing, it was, I told myself, "muscle strain." Muscle strain was a far more accurate diagnosis than I ever imagined. The muscle was my heart.

Luck enters into many events that change lives. In my case, it was going to a different physician. He looked over my medical records and said that my cholesterol was too high. He noted that my father had died of heart disease and my blood pressure was higher than normal, making me a prime candidate for a heart attack. When he asked me about any pain I had in my chest during exercise, I passed it off as indigestion, but he wasn't fooled. He encouraged me to

3

have a treadmill test, where heart monitors record information while exercising. A borderline positive result indicated a need for a thallium stress test, a pair of 25-minute heart scans, the first following an injection of a radioactive isotope and the second after going on the treadmill with more thallium injected when at the maximum heart rate. This stress test compares how the heart's blood supply appears at rest and at peak demand. When enough blood doesn't reach the heart muscles at higher exertion levels, ischemia (ISS-KEEM'-EE-A) results. And I had it.

When the thallium scan proved positive, the next step was an angiogram. I wasn't too keen about this procedure—a catheter is inserted into the femoral artery at the groin and threaded into the heart. Different catheters are used to test heart muscles and valves, and to inject a contrast medium which lets the cardiologist see exactly where any blockages are. The results were worse than expected. My heart's right main artery was 100 percent blocked and the two left arteries were 90 percent and 85 percent obstructed. Polaroid pictures showed me where these blockages were.

I was told there are usually three alternatives. The first is angioplasty, where a balloon is inserted into the heart (in the same manner as an angiogram) and opened to press the obstructing plaque back against the artery walls. Angioplasty wasn't feasible in my case, due to the location and type of blockages. The second alternative was open-heart surgery, a bypass operation, where a section of healthy blood vessel is shunted around each of the blocked coronary arteries. The third alternative was to do nothing except take medication and get my life together so I could die. I was told that if I didn't have a bypass soon, my chances of living another six months were poor.

Here were three doctors, all wanting me to be healthy, telling me I should have a bypass operation and have it soon. I was told that every tick of my heart was like the tick of a time bomb; it could go off at any moment. I couldn't accuse them of having financial motives; I belong to a pre-paid health plan and the bypass wouldn't cost me anything, the doctors would receive no extra payment, and the plan would be some $75,000 poorer. The doctors kept insisting: have a bypass now!

To get them to give me more time to think it over and explore alternatives, I told them I couldn't have the bypass right away because it was against my religion. They asked what religion was that? "I'm a devout coward," I replied.

Scared to death (more accurately, scared *of* death), I started reading everything about heart disease I could get my hands on. I was lucky to be retired, with a background in research and statistical analysis. I had time to search through university libraries and using the Internet, a world-wide computer network, read hundreds of articles in medical journals and books. I found out that there was another alternative to open-heart surgery that I hadn't been told about.

The scientific articles led me to a bestselling book, *Dr. Dean Ornish's Program for Reversing Heart Disease*. This book offers a medically sound and proven alternative. It became my primer for survival, and it remains my guide to this day. Some of what you will read here has its roots in that book and from communications with clinicians and researchers at Dr. Ornish's Preventive Medicine Research Institute. I learned that I can have much more control over my own destiny than I had ever realized. It taught me that my eating habits and lack of aerobic exercise in the past were the reasons for my medical problems today. It explained how to change those habits, to not only stop the progression of heart disease, but how to reverse the damage that I had done to myself. It sounded reasonable, but I was hesitant to make major lifestyle changes on the basis of one book. Especially when my cardiologist and personal physician had doubts about this approach. So I kept on reading.

I found a number of books by Dr. John A. McDougall. These backed up much of what I had learned in Dr. Ornish's book, and went much further in explaining why the changes I should make would help me prevent many other illnesses, improve my general health and even relieve other conditions, such as allergies, I'd had for most of my life. I learned more about what atherosclerosis (hardening of the arteries) is, how it forms, what it looks like and how to treat it.

About this same time, a friend and sailing partner began having severe angina and shortness of breath. He went through the same series of tests that I had, but was told that angioplasty would be helpful. Two days after his angiogram, he had balloon angioplasty to push back the plaque that was blocking his coronary arteries, and a few days later he was home and active again. While I had changed my eating pattern completely, he continued eating the same things as before: meat, cheese, potato chips and cookies with lots of shortening. A few months later he was again suffering severe chest pains and shortness of breath. After more tests he was back in the hospital for a bypass operation. I had given him Ornish's book when his heart problems first started, but it took major surgery before he saw the need to read it. He has come to understand the message and he's now living in a way that makes it unlikely he'll need surgery again. His experience reinforces the danger in putting off lifestyle changes. It's worth your life to begin them as soon as possible.

As I read more about Ornish's program, I learned that one of the important factors for reversing heart disease is being in a support group. I called all the local hospitals, associations and social agencies in the hope of joining one, but there were none in Honolulu. My next step was to convince someone to start one, but the same reply kept coming back: if you want one so badly, why not start one yourself? I called the nearest medical center and met with the persons in charge of health education, who agreed it was a good idea but didn't go ahead with it. After six months of meetings, Kaiser Permanente, Hawaii's largest health maintenance organization, and Castle Medical Center, a preventive-medicine oriented hospital complex, agreed to let me start groups. Suddenly, I was to lead two groups. When we had our first meeting at Castle, an hour-and-a-half drive from my home, the room was swamped with 77 people wanting to join. To take as many as possible, we split into two groups, one in the afternoon and one in the evening. Counting driving time, that made an eight-hour day.

Leading three groups a week and using a great deal of time preparing information, recipes and charts, I found myself spending about 40 hours a week on the *Healing Heart* program. So much for retirement.

To make the support groups available to all who need them, I lead them without cost to the participants or payment for myself. The enthusiasm of the group members and the amazing improvement in health they report have made it a rewarding experience. Members relate they have learned much from our groups, and I have learned much more from them than I could ever have found in books alone. I continue to gain more knowledge and understanding about heart disease, diabetes, arthritis and many other cardiovascular-related diseases. With each new group, I learn new ways how others deal with the adjustment to new and better lifestyles, as well as hints and tips to make those changes easier. This wealth of information is critical to the success of those who seek to improve their health. Each group discovers new and different ways of adapting to a healthier lifestyle.

2

How the Heart Functions

Throughout ancient history, the heart was thought of as the center of our emotions, even the source of thoughts and knowledge. We still say things like good-hearted and cold hearted, and call a story heart rending. Only in the last 1,800 years have the heart's functions been known, and only in the last 200 years has the circulation system been understood.

It is surprising how many people, even those who know they have heart disease or those who had surgery, don't have a clear idea of how the heart works. This non-technical summary may help clarify matters.

Over an average lifetime, counting only the time we are resting, the heart pumps over 50 million gallons of blood— enough to fill four supertankers. If you applied the energy expended in 50 years by an average heart, it could lift over 60,000 tons, the size of a battleship, out of the water. For most of us, the heart beats about 3 million times a year.

Only when the heart malfunctions or stops do we think much about it.

Your heart, which is about the size of your clenched fist, is made up of four chambers, two on the left and two on the right. Each of the two upper chambers is called an *atrium* (both are *atria,* sometimes called *auricles)* and the two lower chambers are called *ventricles* (see fig. 2.1). The atria receive the blood from veins, and the ventricles pump the blood out to the body. The left ventricle, thicker-walled than the right ventricle, sends the blood out to all parts of the body except the lungs. The right ventricle supplies only the lungs with blood. The left and right sides of the heart are separated by a half-inch-thick wall of muscle called the septum. The valves allow blood to flow in only one direction.

When the atria fill with blood from the veins returning to the heart, the valves have higher pressure above than below, and the atria contract, letting blood flow into the ventricles (see fig. 2.3). The filled ventricles then contract and force the blood out through the mitral and tricuspid valves. The aortic and pulmonary valves open and snap shut, letting the blood into the aorta and pulmonary artery. As these valves snap closed, preventing blood from returning to the ventricle, the sound they make (nub-dub, nub-dub) is what we call a heartbeat. This supplies every organ in the body with life-sustaining oxygenated blood, except the heart itself. The coronary arteries are the heart's private circulatory system, fed directly from the aorta. The two main coronary arteries, right and left, branch and divide into smaller and smaller tributaries (see fig. 2.2). Heart muscle would soon die if a main coronary artery became blocked and could not supply enough blood, but the smaller branches are capable of connecting with those of other arteries, providing what is called collateral circulation (see fig. 2.4).

Figure 2.1. Cross-Sectional View of Circulation of Blood Through the Heart

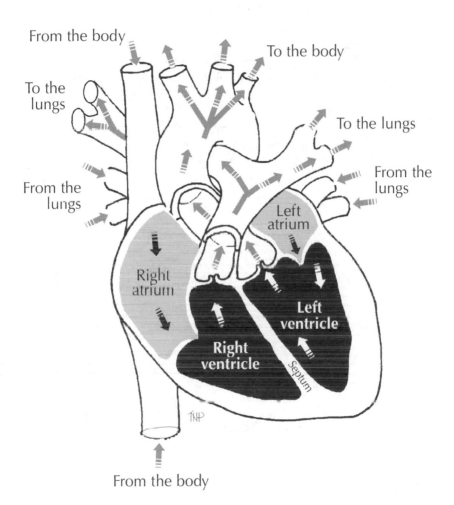

Blood, depleted in oxygen, flows from the veins into the right atrium, then to the right ventricle to be pumped through the pulmonary artery to the lungs. Oxygenated blood from the lungs flows to the left atrium, then to the left ventricle, and is pumped to the aorta and to the body.

Figure 2.2. Coronary Arteries

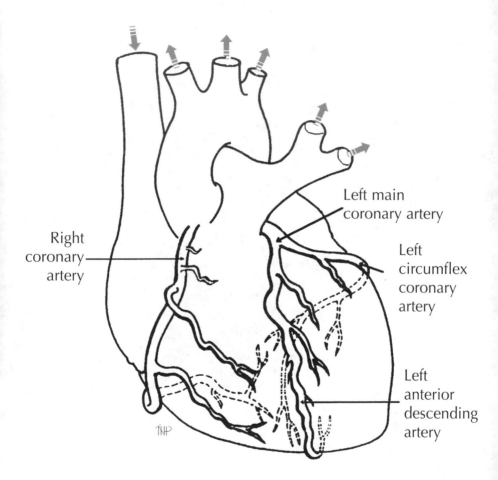

The coronary arteries start from the aorta and spread to many smaller branches that supply the heart muscles. Only the larger arteries are shown here. When plaque blocks these arteries, blood does not reach the muscles. Without oxygenated blood, muscles cannot contract to pump blood.

Figure 2.3. The Heart Valves

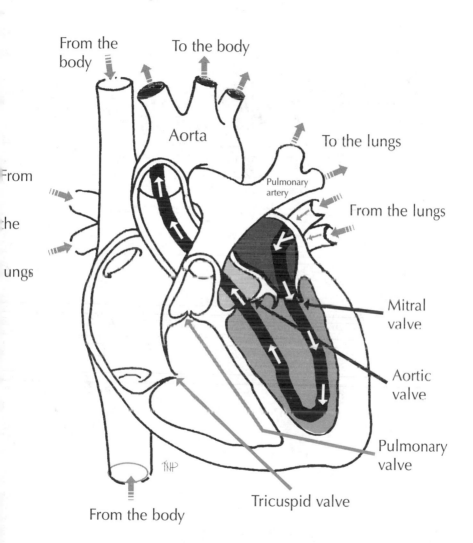

From the body

To the body

Aorta

To the lungs

Pulmonary artery

From the lungs

From

the

ungs

Mitral valve

Aortic valve

Pulmonary valve

Tricuspid valve

From the body

The valves ensure that the blood flows in only one direction. As the muscle contracts to pump the blood out of the chamber, the valve snaps shut, making the sound of the heartbeat.

Figure 2.4. Atherosclerosis

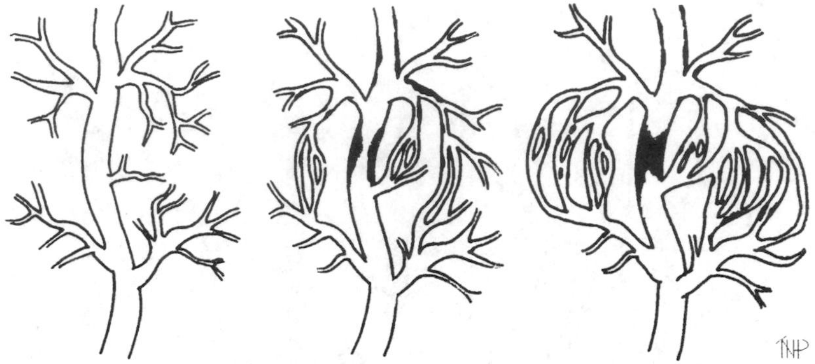

a.   b.   c.

This figure demonstrates atherosclerosis. In part (a), unblocked arteries allow blood to flow without restriction. Next, part (b) shows partly blocked arteries restrict the flow of blood to the muscles, often making an exertion difficult and painful. In some cases *collateral circulation* provides limited relief. Finally, part (c) shows plaque blocking arterial blood flow to heart muscles. Collateral circulation may not be sufficient to keep heart muscles functioning.

3

What Is
Heart Disease?

Heart attacks may strike without warning. In most cases they are the result of a lifetime buildup of plaque, damaging, scarring and eventually blocking the arteries supplying blood to the heart muscles. Knowing what causes plaque is the first step in learning how to reverse it.

Your clenched fist is roughly the size and shape of your heart. If you clench and relax your fist about 60 times a minute, you'll get an idea of what a beating heart looks like. By the time you've done this for a few minutes, you'll have a tired, possibly sore, fist. Imagine tripling the rate of clenching and relaxing to as many as 180 or more times a minute, which is what happens to your heart when you are exercising or running fast. The fist, unlike the heart, isn't made to do that kind of work, and soon you'd have a painful cramp in the muscles you're using, caused by the demand for blood to keep the muscles working which can't be met by the narrow blood vessels supplying them. Many other muscle cramps are cause by a similar shortage of blood.

The heart is basically muscle. Its constant demand for oxygenated blood is supplied by the two large arteries and their branches. When these coronary arteries are clear, the heart muscles can do their job. When there is partial blockage, the arteries provide a supply that may be sufficient to keep the heart muscles working when the activity level is low, but they can't pass the increased flow needed when the demand is much higher—a condition called *ischemia*. Some people are "fortunate" enough to be given a warning when this happens, such as chest pain or other discomfort called *angina*. Many other people will never know that their heart muscle is about to be permanently damaged from lack of enough blood until they suffer a heart attack (technically a *myocardial infarction*). If the damage is only to a small portion of the heart muscle, that portion dies and some scarring occurs, but the heart may continue to function enough to sustain life. If the damage is to a large area, the heart may no longer be able to work as a pump, and the person dies of heart failure.

If a person exercises regularly and eats enough food, there's nothing to worry about, right? Wrong. The problem is in the foods we choose to eat and the kinds of exercise we choose to do.

Americans—and most people in Western industrialized countries—eat a combination of foods that causes most of the health problems they have. The standard American diet (SAD) has more fat and more protein than needed. This diet starts us out on a path to cardiovascular disease before we ever get into our teens. Until the Korean and Vietnam wars, it wasn't realized how bad the situation was. Autopsies of soldiers who died in those wars revealed harmful blockages of the coronary arteries in a majority of these young men, even those younger than 20.

We know that when we eat more fat than we need, we get fatter. But some people eat fatty foods and stay thin, or at least don't become overweight. This may be due to their physical activity level. Some of it is determined by the way their body metabolizes fuel, or can be influenced by the other foods they eat. In most cases, even if they don't get heavier, people who eat high-fat foods are building a foundation for eventual heart disease.

Some fat is present in nearly all foods. Margarine, salad dressings, mayonnaise, nuts, seeds and avocados are very high in fat. All oils are 100 percent fat. When we consume high-fat foods, we are adding more to our system than we usually need for a healthy life. Vegetables, whole grains, beans (legumes) and fruits supply all the fats an adult body needs. The SAD has four times more fat than our body requires and is a major cause of many health problems, especially heart disease.

Most Americans also consume more protein than they need, more calcium than can be absorbed, and too little of the foods that provide basic vitamins and minerals. We aren't very good choosers when it comes to eating. The difference between living a long and full life and being ill or disabled is most often determined by the lifestyle choices we make.

There are other reasons for heart disease besides what we eat. Abusing drugs (alcohol and nicotine are among those drugs) or burning the candle at both ends—not letting our body recover from the abuse we heap on it—also contribute to health problems and a shorter life. These are things we can control through the choices we make.

Many people believe there's nothing they can do about high levels of stress. Changing where we live or where we work is not often a reasonable option. Stressful situations may be difficult to avoid in many parts of our life, but we *can* learn how to deal with stress more effectively. It's possible to live in a stressful world and not be affected by much of it if we learn how to master our reactions to stressful situations.

We can't do anything about our inherited genetic patterns, but we can minimize our own risks. A knowledge of family illnesses can help us to make better choices in our lifestyles.

In the chapters that follow, the mechanisms of heart disease and the choices we can make to prevent and reverse this often fatal condition are explained.

Heart disease can take many forms, but the most common—and the biggest killer of American men and women—is the blockage of the arteries bringing blood to the heart's muscles.

4

The Heart Risk Factor

The bad news is that heart disease is the largest killer of people in the U.S. The good news is that it has become one of the most carefully studied health problems. More is known about the causes and prevention of heart attacks than most other diseases that kill us. That is truly good news, since what has been learned allows us to assess the risks brought about by our lifestyle, and to know what we can do to reduce the risk of dying of heart disease.

Risk factors are odds, something like the chances of winning at a casino. Occasionally someone beats the odds and comes home with a bundle, some others lose every time, but for almost everyone else the odds continue much as predicted.

There are some risk factors you're stuck with. You can't change the genes your parents gave you. Your family's tendency toward heart disease is evaluated from the men who had a heart attack before age 55 and women before 65. These are considered premature heart attacks and may reflect a genetically linked risk. The genes that established your gender, skin color and other physical factors can affect your risk factor. Males have a higher risk than females before age 55, and maintain a 10-year disadvantage compared with women, until age 75 or 80 when the risk equalizes. Black Americans have more high blood pressure and diabetes than other ethnic groups, putting them at higher heart disease risk. Although not yet confirmed, some other genetic factors are suspected of carrying an increased risk of heart disease. Individuals at risk include those who are shorter than average (women under five feet and men under five feet, six inches), men with a bald spot at the top of their head or a receding hairline, and people with a crease across the earlobe. While there's nothing you can do to change these traits, you should keep in mind that if any of these apply to you, the things you *can* do are even more important for you to consider.

The good news continues. The most effective ways to reduce your risk factor are also things you can do something about.

Smoking

Of the 500,000 deaths from coronary artery disease each year, between 20 and 40 percent—100,000 to 200,000—are directly related to smoking tobacco. Quitting smoking cuts the chance of a heart attack by half. But cutting down to fewer cigarettes a day or changing to low-tar, low-nicotine products doesn't do much to reduce the odds. The benefits of quitting start immediately, and between 5 and 10 years after quitting the risk is reduced to the same as for people who never smoked.

Fats

Reducing the amount of fats in what you eat helps clear clogged arteries and helps control cholesterol. The target is to limit fats to no more than 10 percent of the calories eaten. Fats are essential to maintain good health, but Americans typically eat four times more than they need. A balanced diet of vegetables, legumes (beans and lentils), whole grains and fruits will supply all the fats a body requires. Reading labels and avoiding high-fat foods is an insurance policy for health and longevity.

Cholesterol

Keeping fats down, especially saturated fats, is one part of reducing cholesterol. Many foods are high in cholesterol. Reducing the intake of cholesterol-containing foods is crucial. Eggs, meats (including poultry and fish) and dairy products are the main sources of cholesterol. Avoiding them will help reduce blood cholesterol level. Eating high-fiber foods and regular aerobic exercise are also helpful in reducing cholesterol.

When cholesterol is over 200 mg/dl, for each point that cholesterol is lowered, the risk of a heart attack is reduced by 2 percent. For maximum protection against a heart attack, reduce your serum cholesterol level to 150 mg/dl or less. Following the recommendations of *Healing Heart* support groups, the same recommendations as in this book, has helped many people bring their cholesterol levels down from over 300 to below 150 in less than three months.

Blood Pressure

Hypertension is a major contributor to the risk of heart attack and stroke. Every time the diastolic level (the lower number) is reduced one point, the risk of a heart attack is lowered 2 to 3 percent. Reducing fat, animal protein, alcohol and in some cases sodium, as well as taking off excess weight, are some of the ways to reduce blood pressure.

Exercise

The couch potato (someone who gets almost no exercise) is one vegetable that may be harmful to your health. A sedentary lifestyle is favored by more than 60 percent of all Americans, yet it is now known that regular aerobic exercise reduces the risk of heart attack by 35 to 55 percent. This reduction occurs shortly after an individual begins regular exercise. Less strenuous daily activities, like gardening or a walk after dinner, can be beneficial. Regular exercise reduces heart disease risk, lowers blood pressure, helps control weight, can boost "good" HDL cholesterol levels, makes the body's use of insulin more efficient, reduces blood clot formation and makes it easier to control stress. Aerobic exercise combined with some weight training can help keep the body in the best condition to resist disease, and prevent osteoporosis and the effects of aging.

Weight

More than one out of every three Americans is overweight or obese. Overweight people have double the risk of coronary artery disease, and also an increased risk of hypertension, diabetes and high cholesterol. There's also a relationship between what part of the body the fat is on and the risk for heart disease. Waist-heavy people have a higher heart risk than those who accumulate fat around the hips. Regardless of where the fat is, the more overweight a person is, the higher the risk for heart disease.

Diabetes

Over 12 million Americans suffer from adult-onset, non-insulin-dependent diabetes. Men with this condition have two to three times the risk of heart disease, but women increase their heart disease risk from three to seven times. Following the recommendations for preventing and reversing heart disease can also help the body use blood sugars more efficiently, slowing the onset and reducing the severity of diabetes. Many diabetics have been able to reduce and even eliminate the need to inject insulin in just a few weeks. (If you are diabetic and begin this program, be sure to test yourself at least three times a day at the beginning, as demand for insulin drops immediately.)

5

Atherosclerosis

"Hardening of the arteries" is a term many people use for the disease doctors call *atherosclerosis*. The term is a bit deceptive, as it might give the image that the arteries simply harden, like a cooked macaroni noodle after it dries out. It would be more accurate to call this progressive condition "narrowing of the arteries," as this is a closer description of what happens to arteries affected by atherosclerosis.

Excess fats and cholesterol in our blood can irritate the inner lining of the arteries. With the continued intake of the SAD, the arteries begin to change in a more permanent way. The many small injuries attract blood clotting elements (platelets and white blood cells) to repair the damage and stimulate growth of muscle cells, and eventually small scars begin forming inside the arteries. These scars are constantly exposed to blood containing high levels of fat and cholesterol, and they begin to swell. Each individual incident, and there can be hundreds, results in a collection of material called plaque. Plaque, which blocks the flow of blood, is made mostly of cholesterol.

Arteries can also be damaged by trauma from physical injuries or surgery. Prolonged high blood pressure tends to cause injuries. Chemical toxins, such as carbon monoxide and other byproducts of tobacco smoke, as well as factors of some food proteins, can take their toll. Arteries, like most other parts of our body, try to heal themselves. When the irritating effect is not too severe or long-term, healing happens. But when we continue to eat an excess of fats, proteins and toxins typical in the standard American diet, the damage is more than can be fully repaired by the body's natural healing system.

At first the buildup is mostly fat, but as the condition progresses, scars become the main component. These hard, fibrous plaques prevent the artery from remaining flexible, creating what is called "hardening of the arteries." Plaques inside the walls of the arteries restrict the flow of blood to the organs that require it, particularly the heart muscles. Angina (pressure or intense chest pain) is mostly a result of muscles being deprived of blood they need to continue to function. When these muscles don't get enough fuel they can be permanently injured, unable to function again, causing heart failure.

It's important to note that atherosclerosis doesn't just block the arteries to the heart. Blood vessels in the entire body are affected, and major organs can be severely taxed or fail from the lack of sufficient blood.

Plaque formations are doubly dangerous. As the arteries become more brittle, any excess pressure, perhaps from a sudden increase in activity, can rupture the arterial wall and cause an aneurism or a stroke. If these plaque deposits break off, a clot can be sent to the heart and can cause a heart attack, or if it is in the artery feeding the brain, can result in a stroke.

For most people, atherosclerosis can be reversed. It was thought for many years that the damage was always permanent and that the only way to make sure the heart could receive a sufficient blood supply was to repair the arteries through surgery. Unfortunately, many medical professionals still recommend angioplasty or bypass surgery first, rather than giving their patients the choice of reversing their condition through lifestyle changes.

Non-surgical reversal is not indicated for all persons. In those cases where the disease may have progressed too far, surgical intervention may be needed to save life. To be fair, physicians have found that not all persons are willing to make the drastic changes needed to regain a healthy heart. Some patients will promise to follow lifestyle changes, only to abandon them as soon as they begin to feel better. Only consultation with your family physician and a cardiologist can determine what choice is best for you. In most cases, surgery can be put off for a month or two, and in that period a significant improvement can be made by following a program such as the one recommended here.

Unfortunately, the progress of heart disease doesn't stop following angioplasty or a bypass. These procedures allow more blood to flow to the heart, but these repaired or replaced arteries are certain to become blocked again if changes in diet, exercise and dealing with stress are not made. If a person continues the same lifestyle that led to the problem, angioplasty or open-heart surgery will often be needed again.

6

Heart Attack

Knowing the symptoms of a heart attack can mean the difference between life and death. More than 50 percent of the persons having a heart attack wait two hours or more before getting medical assistance, a complication that causes half of them (over 250,000 a year) to die before they get to a hospital.

Possibly many heart attack sufferers don't want to cause a panic for what they think (and hope) is only a minor problem. It's so much more comforting to believe that it is nothing serious, and to keep that river in Egypt, *denial,* flowing through our hopes. A second reason, which may actually account for more of the delayed action, is that most people aren't fully aware of the signs of a heart attack. Movie and TV portrayals, where people grip their chests and fall over, are not quite accurate and may lead people to believe that a heart attack has to resemble that performance. Profuse sweating, dizziness and nausea are common, and an ache or tingling in the shoulders and arms often occurs. Sometimes there's a feeling that something hit the "funnybone" in the elbow. When questioned, most heart attack victims did not know, before they had the attack, where the pain would be and what it would feel like. The common belief was that a heart attack would feel like a knife plunged into the left side of the chest. More often, sufferers reported afterwards that they felt a crushing feeling in the center of the body.

Some common symptoms of a heart attack (myocardial infarction) are:

♥ Feeling of fullness in the chest that lasts two minutes or more.
♥ Intermittent or consistent mild ache or pressure. Can also be a severe squeezing or crushing feeling in the center of the chest or spreading out across the whole chest, up to the neck, jaw, shoulders or down the arms.
♥ Cold sweats, weakness, nausea, vomiting, shortness of breath and fainting.

What happens during a heart attack:
Muscles need constantly renewed oxygen-enriched blood from the lungs. If the supply is cut off or slowed down by blocked or spasming arteries, the muscles cannot keep working. As the blood supply to the heart decreases, muscle cells start dying. A mild heart attack can last up to an hour, possibly causing relatively slight damage. Although any damage usually leaves some scarring, the heart may be able to overcome the effects of these scars and continue its work as a pump. If the damage is greater, large areas of the heart may be destroyed, leading to permanent disability or death. Even moderate heart attacks can cause complications, such as rapid and irregular heart rhythms, affecting how much blood is circulated in the body.

What a doctor or paramedic might do in the case of a heart attack:

An i.v. (a tube that carries medications directly into the blood stream) will usually be placed into a vein in an arm or hand. Oxygen may also be given, usually through a breathing mask. TPA, a specialized clot-dissolving agent, given within the first three hours of the beginning of the attack can rapidly dissolve the clots that cause most heart attacks. When the equipment is available, electronic sensors attached to the chest will monitor the heart's activity (EKG). These will be hooked up to a TV-like monitor, and the medical staff can see how things are progressing both at bedside and from a central location away from the patient. Blood samples will be drawn to check for specific enzymes that are commonly present after a heart attack. The patient may feel ready to get up and walk around, but may be kept immobilized for a while, often the best medical option at the moment.

Avoiding delay in getting medical attention is the most important key to survival. It is far better to call an ambulance or have someone take you to a nearby emergency room than to wait a while to see what happens. Unless your doctor has the proper emergency equipment in the office, going directly to an emergency facility or calling an ambulance may be more life-saving than going to your doctor's office. Just receiving a dose of TPA at the right time may be enough to save a life. Many heart attack victims lose consciousness very suddenly, so driving alone to a hospital may be dangerous to the victim, pedestrians and other drivers.

7

Angiogram

For a person who has never had an angiogram, the thought of making a hole in the groin, putting a tube through it into an artery, and then threading that tube all the way up to the heart can be frightening. Not only can an angiogram sound terrifying, but the worry about what may be discovered is enough to raise anxiety levels even higher.

The procedure, called *coronary angiography,* is usually only ordered after other diagnostic tests show the possibility of heart disease. Although, as in all surgery, there is a risk of complication or even death, it has become more common and safer in recent years. Over 750,000 angiograms are performed each year in the U.S. Complications are rare, and most people suffer no more than a sore groin and a bruise-like discoloration near the entrance site that can last from a few days to a few weeks.

If you become a candidate for an angiogram, most likely you'll be given materials that explain the procedure and possibly a film or video of a person going through the whole procedure. It helps to watch these videos. Also, a description of my experience may give you an idea of what having an angiogram is like. Since every hospital and each doctor may do things a little differently, other persons may have a different experience.

A few days before the angiogram, I had some lab tests done that required drawing a small amount of blood. Though some hospitals have patients come in the night before, my appointment was for 7:30 A.M. on the morning of the catheterization, which was scheduled to begin at 8:00 A.M. I was told not to eat or drink anything except clear liquids, no caffeine or alcohol, after midnight. I was also advised which medications shouldn't be taken for six days before the procedure, and others that shouldn't be taken the morning of the catheterization. I was asked to bring any medications I regularly take and would need following the angiogram in their original containers. I also had to shave the hair on my right groin the night before the angiogram.

I was told I would be able to leave about six hours after the procedure if there were no complications, but I should prepare an overnight bag and something to read or keep me busy just in case. I was cautioned not to drive until the following day, so I arranged for someone to pick me up at the hospital and take me home.

As luck would have it, there was an accident on the freeway on the way to the hospital that backed up traffic for miles. That raised my anxiety level to an all-time high. When I called the hospital to report I'd be late, I found that most of the surgical team was stuck in the same traffic jam, but that didn't help my anxiety. After arriving, I signed all the usual paperwork and went to the catheterization labs where the procedure is done.

Putting on a gown backward, open in the front, can be somewhat embarrassing, but I was the only person who was looking. I was placed on a narrow padded table with machines and monitors all around me. The room was quite cool, but I was covered with a warm blanket while being hooked up to enough wires to make a journey to outer space. The technicians were friendly, explained anything I wanted to know, but were busy getting everything ready. When I told them that I was scared to death, especially after being stuck in a traffic jam, they told me that they usually give patients a small dose of Valium to calm them down. On a monitor I saw my blood pressure was extremely high, but after they added Valium to the i.v. tube, my pressure fell to low normal. I had no feeling of high or low, just a lot less anxiety.

The doctor told me that he didn't have to cut the skin to get into the artery; a small puncture device did that. He said that it might be the only discomfort I'd feel. As I gazed at all the electronic equipment and video monitors, I waited for the pain of the puncture to tell me that the procedure had started, but there was none. Soon I was told to look at the monitor to see the catheter going up the artery into my heart. I hadn't known until then they had begun.

I watched as different tests were performed on my heart's muscles and valves and felt a flush of warmth in my chest when they injected a contrast medium, which lets the X rays display the flow in the smaller arteries of the heart. I could actually watch the blood pulsing through the arteries of my heart. I remember wishing I could save that amazing image, and later I was given some Polaroid photos of it to take home with me. A few minutes later I was transferred to a gurney and wheeled into a recovery room. A firm and steady hand pressed down heavily on my groin.

In the recovery room a nurse placed a sandbag on the puncture site. I got a drink of juice and a small sandwich. I was still hooked up to a number of monitors, including a clip on my toe to see how much oxygen was in my blood.

About a half-hour later, after at least a half-dozen careful evaluations by the recovery room nurses, I was moved into a private room to rest and recover and eat lunch. I recall that after it was over, my strongest feeling was hunger.

About three hours later the cardiologist came by to tell me what he found in the angiogram and to tell me I could go home in another hour. It was far less frightening after I'd been through it. The most difficult part was lying still on my back for four hours, not being able to raise my head or move to either side. When I think back about how scared and nervous I was, it is clear now that it was more a fear of the unknown. Even reading a booklet and watching a video wasn't enough to convince me how smooth and painless it would be. A year later, when I bravely suggested to my doctor that I ought to have another angiogram to show how much my coronary arteries had improved, he told me that it wasn't worth the risks. Although the odds are less than 1 percent, there is a slight chance of a heart attack, stroke, clotting, bleeding or perforation of the heart during an angiogram. The contrast medium also can cause hives, nausea or vomiting. About 1 out of 20 people has some complications—including infection and heart attack—after an angiogram.

The small risks of angiography were worth it to me. Knowing the precise nature of my heart problem, I learned from research studies about my type of blockage and compared it with others. I may have angiography sometime in the future to show how much I've improved by making lifestyle changes, and to demonstrate how effective those changes are. In the meantime, I'll have to be satisfied knowing that I can now exercise strenuously and enjoy life more, without angina or fatigue. My lifestyle changes have made that possible.

8

Angioplasty

——∿—— Opening blocked arteries without major surgery was first performed by a technique called *angioplasty* in 1977. Only ten years later, nearly 250,000 of these procedures had been performed.

Beginning like an angiogram, balloon angioplasty uses a special catheter with a balloon-like bladder at the tip that is filled with a fluid and then expanded when it is at the site of a blockage. Unlike the angiogram, where the patient can follow much of what is happening, in angioplasty most patients do not see the procedure. The principle is quite simple: if pressure can push the plaque back against the artery walls, the obstruction can be made smaller and the blood can pass through more easily (see fig. 8.1).

Unfortunately, nature doesn't always respond the way we would like it to. In some cases, the plaque deposits re-form almost at once, creating the same blockage. In some cases the problem becomes worse. In nine out of ten cases, arteries will have increased flow, but within three years, more than 60 percent of these procedures will have to be redone, 40 percent with another angioplasty and 22 percent with bypass surgery. Blockages may also begin forming in new locations. If the causes of the problem (usually related to diet, lack of exercise and smoking) are not altered, angioplasty is likely to only provide temporary relief of more serious problems.

Angioplasty relieves chest pain for half to three-quarters of the people who undergo it, but the risks and complications are much greater than those for an angiogram. While only a very few people, about one-tenth of 1 percent, die from complications of angioplasty, because of the chance of complications, a cardiac surgeon prepared to perform immediate open-heart surgery will usually be present. Between 3 and 5 percent of angioplasty patients will require immediate bypass surgery. However, the application of anti-clotting agents during angioplasty has brought about an improved success rate.

There are variations of balloon catheterization that use *laser beams* to melt the plaque deposits and *stents* (a framework support, about the size of a ballpoint pen spring) to keep the artery open. Stents are usually considered temporary, giving a person time to have surgery later.

Atherectomy is another procedure. It involves a high-speed shaving device, or fine abrasive head, that pares the plaque off in very fine layers from the inside. Sometimes called "Roto-Rooters," these work in much the same way as sewer-pipe cleaners. The risk factors in laser and atherectomy procedures are higher than for balloon angioplasty.

Figure 8.1. Angioplasty

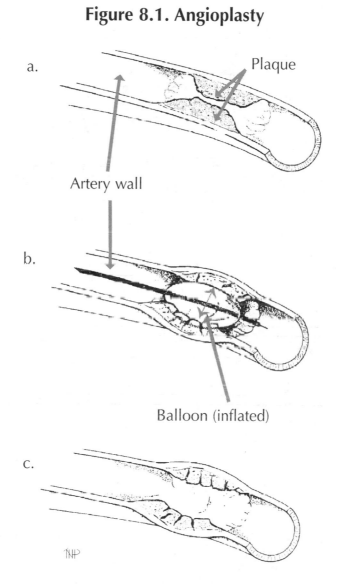

a. Artery partially blocked with plaque.
b. Balloon catheter inserted and inflated.
c. Artery immediately following compression of plaque.

9

Coronary Bypass (Open-Heart) Surgery

─╰─ When the heart's arteries are blocked to a degree where it becomes difficult, sometimes even impossible, to continue normal activity, bypass surgery may be recommended. In a bypass operation, additional arteries, normally made from leg veins, are used to detour around (bypass) the blocked arteries. Usually the patient is able to gradually resume normal activities after a short recuperation period. This procedure doesn't open the blocked arteries, and it does nothing to reverse the buildup of plaque that clogs the arteries. It only provides an alternate route for blood to reach the heart muscles. In many cases, surgery is the only choice when the blockage is so severe that the danger of heart failure is too great to try any other alternative. For such people, the operation is truly a life saver. For a great many others, there may be other alternatives.

Physicians and surgeons have seen the improvement that bypass surgery offers many patients. They have also seen

41

patients opt for lifestyle changes that include serious dietary changes and aerobic exercise, only to watch these patients gradually lapse back to their old eating habits and sedentary ways. Sooner or later such lapses result in the need for surgery, if a heart attack does not come first. A doctor may press for an operation because the outcome of surgery is more certain than promises and good intentions. If bypass surgery has been recommended, it may be the only reasonable choice, but in many cases, such as mine, there may be less drastic options available. Following lifestyle recommendations such as those in this book may bring about a reversal of coronary artery blockage. Before making a final decision, I recommend that you read *Dr. Dean Ornish's Program for Reversing Heart Disease* and discuss his suggested alternatives with your doctors and family.

Although surgeons and hospitals have slight variations in their procedures, the typical bypass operation starts in the morning with the patient receiving a tranquilizer to help calm the anxiety usually found before any operation. Local anesthesia is given and i.v. feeds are inserted in the arm or wrist to allow the administration of fluids, medications and anesthesia. Other i.v. lines are used to measure oxygen content and pressure of the blood, and to place medications directly into the heart. A special catheter will be placed in a neck vein and pushed down into the heart to provide measures of heart function through pressure and temperature. Another catheter will be placed into the bladder to measure kidney function and blood supply. A combination of drugs is fed into the i.v. to relax muscles, make the patient drowsy (which prevents the patient from suddenly moving during the operation) and to block pain. Two tubes are inserted down the throat, one into the windpipe connected to the respirator to take over the job of breathing, and the other to collect stomach fluids and prevent nausea. An anticoagulant drug such as *Heparin* is given to help prevent clots and strokes. At the end of the operation, a drug will be given to reverse the effect of the anticoagulant.

When the surgeons are ready to open the chest, an incision is made down the sternum (the midline of the breastbone) and retractors slowly separate the chest opening, revealing the lungs and the pericardium, the tough sac that protects the heart. While this is being done, another surgical team is removing sections of vein, each about eight-inches long, from a leg. The heart sac is opened and the heart-lung machine is connected. When the heart-lung machine has taken over the pumping and oxygenation, the bypass procedure begins.

The aorta is clamped shut and the heart is stopped and then cooled. For each of the arteries to be bypassed, a hole is made in the aorta and one end of a leg vein is attached to the aorta. The other end is connected to a place below the blockage in the coronary artery. In some cases, the internal mammary artery, just above the aorta, is used as the source of the bypass supply. When the bypasses are completed, the heart is gradually returned to normal temperature and the aorta is unclamped. At this point the heart either starts on its own, or an electrical shock is given to start it again. As the heart begins circulating the blood on its own, the heart-lung machine is disconnected. Before the chest is closed, the surgeons make sure the splices are sealed and there is no bleeding.

More than 500,000 bypass operations are performed every year in the U.S. alone. Of these, many patents will become candidates for a second, and sometimes a third bypass operation. It is important to understand that the original cause of the problem is not changed by this surgery. If lifestyle patterns that fostered the problem are not changed, coronary artery disease will continue to threaten the patient's life.

In *McDougall's Medicine, A Challenging Second Opinion*, a comparison of the risks and benefits of lifestyle changes, angioplasty and bypass surgery are given. Some of the factors, updated since this book was published, are:

Table 9.1. Risks from Lifestyle Changes, Angioplasty and Bypass Surgery

Factor	Lifestyle	Angioplasty	Bypass
Early artery reclosure	none	30%	20%
Atherosclerosis stopped, slowed or reversed	yes	no	no
Brain dysfunction	none	none	15%
Blood transfusions	none	none	likely
Heart attack (during)	none	5%	5%
Complications (during)	none	10%	13%
Death (elderly, during)	none	1%	2%
Cost in dollars (1996)	none	10,000–35,000	50,000–80,000

In addition to the cost of the operations, time off from work, stress to the family and risk factors also need to be considered.

Figure 9.1. Coronary Artery Bypass

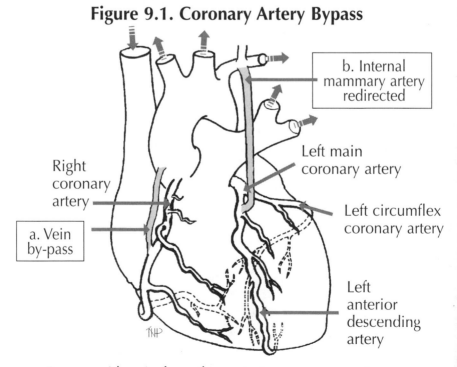

a. Bypass with vein from the aorta to a coronary artery.
b. Internal mammary artery bypass to a coronary artery.

10

Cholesterol

Present in the tissue of all animals, cholesterol is needed by the body as a structural element in all cell membranes, a building block for some hormones and many other important functions. Problems develop when people have too much of this white, fat like waxy material. The liver and other organs of most people produce between 500 and 1,000 milligrams of cholesterol a day, which is usually more than the body needs. The extra amount is filtered out. Adding cholesterol in our diet is seldom necessary.

All animal products contain cholesterol. When meat, fish, fowl, eggs or dairy products are eaten, additional cholesterol is added to that which we make ourselves, and often this is more than the body's cholesterol filtering system can eliminate.

Scientists are not in complete agreement about how cholesterol circulates through our body, but they believe the liver makes bubbles of proteins combined with triglycerides (fats) and cholesterol, called lipoproteins. *Very low density lipoprotein* (VLDL), the largest of these, deposits triglycerides in fat cells and muscles, to be stored until they are needed. When the VLDL releases triglycerides, the bubble becomes smaller and then carries the cholesterol to the cells for metabolism. This smaller cell changes to a *low density lipoprotein* (LDL). LDL is often called "bad" cholesterol, since it adds to the total cholesterol already in the bloodstream. When there is more cholesterol than is needed by the cells, the liver's LDL receptors try to filter it out in order to excrete it as waste. Saturated fats can prevent these LDL receptors from doing their job. Often more cholesterol exists than can possibly be filtered and eliminated, and it circulates in the bloodstream, eventually accumulating on the walls of the arteries. These accumulations build up small nodules, called *plaque,* that obstruct the flow of blood. More information about this buildup can be found in Chapter 5 Atherosclerosis.

The liver also makes a *high density lipoprotein* (HDL), which holds less cholesterol than the LDL. When this circulates it can pick up cholesterol and bring it back to the liver, where some of it is filtered and eliminated. HDL is often called "good" cholesterol, since it can be beneficial in lowering the total cholesterol in the blood. Exercise can be helpful in raising HDL "good" cholesterol.

The cholesterol you get from what you eat, made outside your body, is never "good" cholesterol. When you consume foods that have cholesterol, which can only come from animal products, you are increasing the chance of forming plaque and clogging your arteries. Saturated fats can interfere with the process that filters and eliminates cholesterol, thereby increasing the cholesterol level in your body. Fats are explained in more detail in another section..

Studies of people in two countries illustrate how what we eat can affect cholesterol. In China, a wide, scientifically selected sample from every single county, a total of 6,500 people, has been under examination since 1983. Their food intake and life habits have been carefully logged, and they have been subjected to many medical diagnostic tests. The typical Chinese person eats very little animal protein or saturated fats. The usual cholesterol levels for Chinese people (average 88-165) are lower than for Americans (average 155-274), and coronary heart disease is rare among Chinese. Death from colon cancer is also extremely low. The Japanese, who traditionally consume very low levels of saturated fats, have the lowest levels of cholesterol and heart disease of all industrialized countries.

Compare this with Finland, which has the highest consumption of saturated fats, the highest cholesterol levels and the highest rate of heart disease. The U.S. diet is only slightly less rich than the Finnish diet, and we have the second highest rate of heart disease.

Lowering cholesterol is best accomplished by changing the foods you eat. Eliminating saturated fats and reducing the cholesterol in your diet are both important to good health. Dr. Ornish, in his heart disease reversal program, recommends eating foods with no more than five milligrams of cholesterol a day, a small glass of non-fat milk or a four-ounce serving of fat-free yogurt. Even that small amount may make it difficult for you to bring your cholesterol level below 150 mg/dl, where it needs to be to begin reversing the damage already caused in your arteries. It was once thought that anything under 200 mg/dl was a safe cholesterol level, and many physicians and health foundations are still satisfied with that number, but more recent research shows the reversal process improves and the risk of heart attack lowers most when the cholesterol level is below 150. When your cholesterol level is above 200, for every point it is reduced, the risk of heart attack is lowered by 2 percent.

For people in good health with no family history of heart disease or other risk factors, consuming foods with small amounts of cholesterol may pose no immediate danger. But those with an elevated risk of heart disease should avoid dietary cholesterol. Since saturated fats prevent the body from removing excess cholesterol, these also should be reduced or eliminated. A national consumer education organization warned that a medium-size bag of buttered popcorn sold at movie theaters may have more saturated fat than a breakfast of bacon and eggs, a large hamburger with french fries for lunch and a steak dinner with all the trimmings. Sound impossible? Movie theater popcorn is typically popped in coconut or palm oil, extremely high in saturated fat.

Other things can be done to lower cholesterol in addition to watching what you eat. An important benefit will likely happen automatically to most people when they follow a proper diet and take off a few pounds. Being overweight leads to higher LDL and total cholesterol. Most people find that for every two pounds of excess fat that is lost, one point (mg/dl) of total cholesterol is also lost. Just losing 20 pounds will likely reduce your cholesterol by ten points. In *Healing Heart* support groups, most overweight people who followed the diet faithfully and who started a moderate exercise program lost an average of over two pounds a week for the first ten weeks—and they kept it off. When your body reaches the weight that is best for you, you should still be able to eat all you want of the proper foods, without counting calories, and remain at that weight.

Exercise is important in reducing cholesterol. A daily program of aerobic exercise will help you to lower and keep down your cholesterol level. As you exercise aerobically, your blood pumps through the arteries at a higher rate, and the high density lipoproteins (HDL) can carry more cholesterol away. Doing aerobic exercise for at least 40 minutes a day, at least five days a week, is needed to get maximum benefits in reversing heart disease and lowering risk.

Cholesterol-lowering medications are commonly recommended.

If prescribed by your physician, continue to take them as directed. As you follow all the elements recommended in this book and your cholesterol goes down, your doctor may wish to gradually lower the dosage of some medications. Many *Healing Heart* support group participants are able to stop taking their medications completely after a short while. Don't alter your medications on your own; always discuss any change you may want to make with your doctor. If your physician doesn't want you to reduce the medication, ask why. If the answer doesn't satisfy you, it is better to look for a different doctor than to keep the same one and ignore the advice given.

Some over-the-counter preparations claim to reduce cholesterol, and they may possibly help, though there are often unwanted side effects. Psyllium-based supplements, for example, can cause some people to have diarrhea, stomach cramps and a bloated feeling. Using psyllium instead of eating fiber-rich foods can cause some people to depend on a daily dose to keep their bowels moving normally. Psyllium is mostly dietary fiber, but a low-fat vegetarian diet will give you all the fiber you need to both reduce cholesterol and maintain normal bowel function.

Testing blood for cholesterol is simple and inexpensive. The most accurate measure comes from blood drawn by a professional laboratory and analyzed with constantly recalibrated equipment operated by skilled technicians. The finger pin-prick tests are only as accurate as the equipment and skill of the person administering it. Since these portable machines are moved from place to place, they require more frequent calibration and adjustment, which is not always done. When you are having your cholesterol measured, don't exercise for at least two hours before the test, as exercise can temporarily elevate cholesterol levels. Illness, pregnancy, some medications and recent surgery can also influence blood cholesterol levels. If your test measures LDL or triglycerides, you should not eat or drink anything (except water) for at least 14 hours before the blood is drawn. Always call ahead to see if LDL or triglycerides are to be tested.

When the results come back, make sure you get the exact number of all the measurements. You can use the chart in Appendix H to record them. Don't be satisfied with being told "Your cholesterol is normal" or "You're okay." Reversing heart disease means maintaining levels of cholesterol much lower than what is "normal" for others.

One of the figures you may be given is a risk factor ratio. This is usually the total cholesterol divided by the HDL. This ratio, according to your age and sex, can give an indication of the risk of dying from heart disease.

Table 10.1. Risk Factor Ratio

Risk factor (Total/HDL)	Men's Ratio	Women's Ratio
Very low (half of average)	under 3.0	under 3.3
Low	4.0	3.8
Average	5.0	4.5
Moderate (2 times average)	9.5	7.0
High (3 times average)	23.0 +	11.0 +

For years we've been hearing the advice to eat chicken or fish instead of beef, pork or lamb. What is hard for many people to accept is that the leaner the meat, the more cholesterol it contains. Each ounce of lean beef will have between 20 and 25 milligrams of cholesterol, depending on the cut, but an ounce of lean skinless chicken can have more than beef, often as much as 25 milligrams. An ounce of dark turkey meat contains 32 milligrams of cholesterol, and fish contains between 10 to over 100 milligrams of cholesterol per ounce (sometimes five times that of steak). All animal products contain cholesterol, but no plant foods have measurable amounts of cholesterol.

Physicians at the Weimar Institute have determined that

the average American male eats foods containing about 500 milligrams of cholesterol a day, about the same amount as his body makes internally. The typical American female eats about 350 milligrams of cholesterol. Not one milligram of that is needed by the body, which makes all it needs.

Vegans, strict vegetarians who eat no dairy or egg products, consume no cholesterol in their diet. Numerous studies show that vegetarians live longer and have fewer heart attacks and fewer incidences of coronary artery disease, diabetes and many types of cancer than the general population—the meat eaters. Many studies estimate that 70 percent of these diseases can be prevented with changes in eating habits.

Much of what follows in this book will explain how to reduce cholesterol and establish a lifestyle for optimum health.

11

You Are
What You Eat

Before I learned I had heart disease, I didn't pay a great deal of attention to nutrition. I had heard it was better to use margarine than butter, better to use olive oil or canola oil than lard, and better to eat chicken than beef. I ate what was supposed to be "better" and I still got heart disease.

I found out that doctors typically aren't given much training in nutrition and that some so-called nutrition experts are not well qualified in that field. A large sample of physicians was asked how much nutrition training they received in medical school. The average was less than three hours, with many having only one hour or less. That's out of nearly 3,500 hours of medical training. The truth is that doctors may get their nutrition information from the same newspapers and TV programs we do, and unless they have taken extra training in nutrition, they may not know much more about nutrition than the rest of us.

Some physicians have studied how foods and supplements affect our health. They have found that what we eat is an essential factor in our ability to resist and reverse many diseases and other health problems. Interestingly, these doctors are not the first to tell us this. Throughout the past 5,000 years, important writers have said much the same thing and have been largely ridiculed or ignored, just like many of those saying it today.

This may have something to do with our reluctance to take responsibility for our own health rather than let it fall to someone else. Physicians care about our health, but we are only one of a number of patients. Most doctors cannot possibly be as involved in each patient's personal situation as each of us can and should be about our own health. We have the power to control a major part of our own destiny. What we put into our body and how we use or abuse our body may be the single most important factor deciding how long we live and how well we will be while we are alive.

There are many mistaken beliefs about nutrition. Some may sound threatening to persons who have been advised to eliminate animal products and fat from their diet. Often heard are remarks about how vegetarians don't get enough calcium, proteins, essential amino acids, vitamins and minerals. These beliefs are not based on scientific studies or established nutritional information. Some are based on advertising campaigns, such as "Milk does a body good" and "Where's the beef?" Others may simply be from a lack of knowledge. The U.S. Department of Agriculture's (USDA) current food pyramid is the result of enormous pressure from meat producers and the many special interest groups attempting to increase consumption of meat, poultry and dairy products. Even the concerted effort of one of the nation's most powerful lobbies, however, could not prevent the truth from being released in January 1996 when the new USDA Dietary Guidelines finally admitted, "A vegetarian lifestyle is quite consistent with good health." The American Dietetic Association, a national organization of nutrition and diet information specialists, has issued a policy statement on vegetarian diets. The ADA is not a vegetarian group, and the majority of its members are not vegetarians, so it cannot be considered a biased view. The complete document is in Appendix G of this book. This authoritative resource should set straight many mistaken beliefs and provide answers to many questions about this recommended healthy lifestyle.

AN INSPIRATIONAL EXAMPLE: DR. RUTH HEIDRICH

More than a dozen years ago, at age 47 and with a successful career, Ruth was diagnosed with breast cancer. After losing both breasts and facing painful chemotherapy and radiation treatments, she was advised by Dr. John McDougall to change her diet and lifestyle instead. Since then she has followed a nutritional plan that is essentially the same as the recommendations given in this book. She consumes 10 percent calories from fat, 10 percent from protein and the rest from complex carbohydrates. For over 14 years she has eaten no meat, fish, poultry, dairy, egg products or white sugar. Now past 60, she has won, in her class, over 44 marathons world-wide and 6 First Place trophies from the Ironman Triathlon, considered by some to be the most grueling race in the world. She still competes in about 50 races a year, takes first place in her class in most of them, and yet she takes no vitamins or supplements. Her regular checkups show no deficiencies, and her cancer has not spread to any other part of her body. When people say that they can't get enough energy or can't receive all their nutritional requirements from a low-fat vegetarian diet, Dr. Heidrich's example is living proof that we can. Her book *A Race for Life* is an inspirational story of her victory over cancer.

Understanding the reasons for avoiding certain foods should make it easier to give them up, or at least easier to reduce the quantity eaten. There are many dietary considerations for maintaining good health and reducing the risk of disease or early death. Knowledge about fats, carbohydrates, protein and cholesterol is essential for a healthy heart. Knowing what to eat and what to avoid will help you make the proper choices for a longer, healthier life. Before examining the most important nutritional factors for a healthy heart, here is some information about things we put in our body:

Sodium is often blamed for high blood pressure and other health problems. Although there is clear evidence that excess sodium can affect blood pressure and result in heart disease and other health problems, only a small percentage of the population is sodium sensitive, with a definite link between even small amounts of salt intake and their blood pressure. Others can eat moderate amounts of salt with no problem. There is no blood test or laboratory procedure to see if you are one of the few who must carefully limit salt, but you can try this out for yourself. First, if your blood pressure is normal and you currently eat salty foods (which means most prepackaged foods), you don't need to test yourself. If you have hypertension and want to see if you are sodium sensitive, you can try the following: For a period of 10 days, avoid all forms of food with salt or added sodium (you'll get all the sodium your body needs from other food sources). Read labels carefully and avoid canned or processed foods. Once each day, at about the same time of day, take your blood pressure. Write it down where you can find it every day, perhaps on a calendar. If you can't take your own blood pressure or get someone to do it, many localities have walk-in clinics (and often fire stations) that will take your blood pressure without charge. Avoid machines in drugstores, as they are not always calibrated regularly and may give inaccurate readings. After the 10-day sodium fast, begin eating moderate amounts of foods containing sodium. It isn't necessary to heap salt on; just eat foods that have a higher sodium content. Continue your daily blood pressure measurement for the next 10 days. It may take a week or so to see any change, but if you see the numbers rising for three days, stop the test. You'll then know that your blood pressure is influenced by salt. If there was no change in blood pressure during the 10 days of salt intake, it would indicate you're not presently sodium sensitive. Different medications, age and other physical conditions can change your sensitivity, so don't overdo your salt intake and continue to check your blood pressure at regular intervals, at least twice a year.

High levels of sodium, including table salt, are a common ingredient in processed foods and many restaurant dishes. The typical American eats three times more sodium than the *maximum* recommended daily intake of 2,400 milligrams. This can lead to kidney failure and to heart attacks and stroke, even for those who are not sodium sensitive. Many foods that don't taste "salty" may be high in sodium, and it is wise to know which these are. Most canned foods, fast-food sandwiches and packaged soups and mixes contain as much as 1,000 to 2,000 milligrams of sodium per serving. A tablespoon of soy sauce has up to 1,300 milligrams, and a typical serving of pizza between 500 and 1,000 milligrams. Many cheeses have between 200 and 300 milligrams per ounce. Commercially packaged bread can have 100 to 300 milligrams per slice. A teaspoon of table salt contains 2,300 milligrams of sodium, far more than is needed for an entire day's intake. Most fresh and frozen vegetables, fruits and whole grains are very low in sodium.

If a recipe calls for salt, see if you can leave it out until the food is on the table, and then lightly sprinkle the surface with a small amount of salt. You'll find you can use much less salt than the recipe calls for and get a saltier taste. Salt added in cooking often makes foods tougher, and much of the taste is lost. Salt substitutes, including "lite salt," which is half potassium chloride, can reduce your sodium intake. Citrus acid is often called "sour salt." When added in very small amounts it can impart a salty flavor—but in larger amounts it can be very sour. Most health food stores carry Bragg's Liquid Aminos, a product made entirely from soybeans. It has a very salty soy sauce flavor but has less sodium. For soy sauce, shoyu or tamari, always use the salt-reduced versions.

Caffeine is one of the world's most popular drugs. It is believed to be harmful to those who already have heart disease and many other health problems, but the link has not been fully evaluated. Caffeine can shorten reaction time, keep one awake temporarily and give the feeling of increased energy. As with many drugs, the body can build a tolerance to caffeine. This means that a person may need increasing amounts to get the same effects. As the dosage increases, trembling, muscle tension, irritability, nervousness, depression, disorientation, lethargy and throbbing headaches can result. For those with little or no tolerance, a single cup of coffee may produce some of these symptoms. Others, whose body has become used to the drug, may be able to drink more than three or four cups of coffee without experiencing any outward signs. Inwardly, blood pressure, cholesterol, heart and metabolic rates, respiration and blood glucose concentration are all affected by caffeine. While some studies claim to have linked caffeine to cancer, benign breast fibrocystic disease and other illnesses, the evidence is not sufficient to link any of these with certainty.

Table 11.1. Common Sources of Caffeine

Source	Serving Size	Caffeine (mg)
Brewed coffee	5-ounce cup	60-150
Instant coffee	5-ounce cup	40-105
Decaffeinated coffee	5-ounce cup	2-5
Strong tea (steeped 5 min)	5-ounce cup	40-100
Weak tea (steeped 3 min)	5-ounce cup	20-50
Cocoa	5-ounce cup	2-10
Coca-Cola	12-ounce can	45
Milk chocolate	2 ounces	2-30
Anacin, Empirin, Midol	2 tablets	65
Excedrin	2 tablets	130
Aqua-Ban, Dexatrim, No-Doz	2 tablets	200

However, persons who have had recent heart surgery or have an irregular heartbeat should definitely avoid caffeine.

Caffeine is a powerful drug and it may be difficult to give up at first. Some people suffer headaches and other discomfort when suddenly discontinuing caffeine. It is usually easier to gradually reduce caffeine than to stop all at once. If coffee is your primary source of caffeine, after your first cup in the morning, mix regular coffee with decaffeinated coffee. Start with about 75 percent regular coffee and reduce the amount after a few days until you are drinking 100 percent decaffeinated coffee. Then gradually do the same for your first cup of the day.

Ruth Heidrich's *Race for Life Cookbook* recommends "Morning Toffee" as a breakfast drink: one teaspoon of *blackstrap* molasses in a cup of hot water. Brimming with vitamins and minerals, it has only 15 calories. I drink it most mornings and find it delicious.

Alcohol is another drug whose effect on heart disease and health has been debated, though the exact degree of cause-and-effect is not clearly established. Excess alcohol is definitely known to be linked to increased risks of cancers of the mouth, larynx, esophagus and pharynx. A relationship between alcohol consumption and cancers of the pancreas, rectum and breast has also been shown. Liver disease is a common result of long-term alcohol use. Some studies have shown a link between small amounts of alcohol and a rise in one kind of HDL "good" cholesterol, but that may not actually reduce total cholesterol.

For many, keeping the amount of alcohol at the low levels is difficult or impossible. Consumption of alcohol in larger amounts can lower HDL, raise blood pressure, damage the heart and also lead to loss of bone mass, which can increase the risk of osteoporosis. It is recommended that persons with increased risk of heart disease avoid excess alcohol. If you choose to drink, you should have no more than two mixed drinks, or two 12-ounce servings of beer, or two 4-ounce glasses of wine a day, preferably with meals.

A 10-year government research project in Denmark, known as the Copenhagen Study, revealed that the consumption of moderate amounts of red wine with meals significantly lowered heart attacks and deaths from heart disease. Those who drank red wine with their meals had 30 percent fewer heart-related deaths than the persons who drank no wine with meals. Binge drinking (at parties or on weekends, rather than drinking regularly with meals) and consuming any quantity of hard liquor did not result in any benefits.

Charcoal-broiled foods have been linked to cancer, but it is primarily the fats that drop onto the coals when meats are cooked that are thought to make the smoke dangerous. Burnt meat and some other foods may also be carcinogenic (can lead to cancer). Barbecuing vegetables does not carry the same risk as with meats if the charcoal has not been used to cook meat.

Vitamins are substances not normally produced in the body that are required for proper cell metabolism. The amounts we need are very small and are found in the foods we eat. With certain exceptions, vitamin supplements are seldom needed. Unfortunately, that's not what most people have been led to believe. Nearly 4 out of every 10 persons in the U.S. take vitamin pills. There is no evidence that taking these vitamin supplements has any positive effect on the length of time we live or on normal physical or sexual performance. There may be little or no harm in taking most normal "one-each-day" dosages of vitamin supplements. If you choose to take a daily multivitamin, do not take "megadose" formulas. Men should avoid multivitamins containing iron. The greatest benefits of vitamins, however, go primarily to those who make and sell them.

Advertisers tell us Americans do not consume enough of the vitamins we need, but those who do *not* take supplements almost never experience effects of vitamin deficiencies (scurvy, pellagra, night blindness, beriberi, etc.) The Recommended Daily Allowances (RDA) were set at very high levels, well in excess of what most persons need, to provide a margin of safety. Makers of vitamin supplements use the RDA figures to instill a fear that we may not be getting enough of these vitamins from our foods, but almost all medical and nutritional professional organizations agree that these supplements are not needed for persons eating a well-balanced diet.

One exception, for people who eat no animal products, is vitamin B_{12} (cobalamin), the only vitamin not available from plant foods. When a person stops eating animal products, at least a five-year supply of B_{12} is usually stored in the body. B_{12} can be supplied by a number of fortified breakfast cereals, some special nutritional yeasts or from B_{12} tablets. A few micrograms (millionths of a gram) daily are all that is needed. However, even among lifelong vegans (vegetarians who use no animal byproducts, including egg or dairy), B_{12} deficiency is extremely rare.

There is some evidence that vitamin E may help reduce the risk of heart attacks. While there is no consensus on the benefits of vitamin E, there seems to be common agreement that taking up to 400 international units (IU) a day may be beneficial and would not be harmful to most people. If later research confirms these preliminary findings, persons with high heart risk will have gained those benefits. Vitamin E is an antioxidant and is also thought to be helpful in preventing some kinds of cancer. Some evidence indicates that antioxidants work better in combinations, such as vitamin C, beta carotene and vitamin E together. Vitamin E comes in capsules, tablets and soft-gels, small gelatin balls containing the liquid vitamin, allowing it to be absorbed rapidly. The gelatin in soft-gels and capsules is most often made from animal products, and for that reason many vegetarians prefer vitamins in tablet form.

Minerals are inorganic compounds (not containing carbon) that make up the major part of the earth's surface. Minerals are absorbed by plants from the soil and water and then become part of the foods we eat. Of the more than 60 minerals present in the human body, only 22 are considered essential.

Minerals make up about 4 percent of our total body weight. A 150-pound person's body has about 6 pounds of minerals, some present in very small amounts. The body needs only about four ten-millionths part of iodine, but calcium needs to be present in nearly two-hundredths part. Although mineral deficiencies are uncommon, without proper nutrition three minerals may be lacking in some people. Additional calcium, present in green leafy vegetables and animal products, may be needed if too much protein has been ingested. Iron, present in peas, beans, green leafy vegetables, nuts and whole and enriched grains, as well as in red meats, is needed for blood. Zinc, present in whole wheat, meats, shellfish and eggs, is needed to heal wounds, for sexual development and to help keep our senses of taste and smell sharp. Iodine deficiency used to be common, causing goiter and thyroid gland problems. In the past 70 years, iodized salt has supplied all the iodine the body needs, amounting to about a half-teaspoon of salt a day from all sources. Much of that iodine comes from salt in processed foods.

Mineral supplements are also touted as a way to prevent and cure disease and live longer, but as is true for vitamins, all the minerals we need are well provided for when we eat a balanced diet. Some makers claim that chelated minerals, those bound to a metallic substance, provide better absorption and are better utilized, but there is no evidence that these are any more useful than any other type of supplement. Don't be led to buy these supplements by high pressure sales claims.

Mineral and vitamin supplements are a high-profit, billion-dollar industry. Supplement distributors take advantage of the feeling many people have that they are not getting adequate nutrition from the foods they consume. For people who get most of their meals from fast-food chains or junk foods, this is probably true. Nutritionists, physicians and medical researchers generally agree that healthy people eating a balanced diet of whole grains, vegetables, legumes and fruits do not need mineral or multivitamin supplements. Taking vitamin and mineral supplements provides some people with a false feeling of security that leads them to be less careful about what they eat.

Fiber is essential in reducing the risk of some kinds of cancer, intestinal disease, gallstones, diabetes, obesity and heart disease. There are two types of fiber. Sponge-like *insoluble* fiber, from grains, legumes, fruits and the outer surface of some seeds, promotes food passage and adds bulk, which reduces food craving. Processed grains and foods often have most of their fiber removed. Use whole grains, brown rice and unprocessed foods to assure sufficient fiber intake.

Whole wheat bread and brown rice have three times the fiber of white bread and white rice. *Soluble* fiber acts as a filter to help prevent some substances, including cholesterol and glucose, from being absorbed into the blood. It also acts as a stool softener, preventing constipation, which is related to colon cancer and diverticulosis. Constipation often leads to straining to clear the bowels, a common precursor of strokes. Paramedics and emergency medical professionals report that one of the most common places that strokes occur is on the toilet. Eating foods high in fiber may help prevent these problems and reduce cholesterol as well.

Refined and processed fruits and juices may also be low in fiber. Comparing an orange and an eight-ounce glass of reconstituted frozen orange juice, the juice has 0.848 grams of fiber while the orange has 9.790 grams, more than 11 times the fiber in the juice. A fresh orange also has a third fewer calories than a glass of orange juice. A few juices do contain high amounts of fiber; unfiltered carrot juice has about 75 percent of the fiber of raw carrots, and tomato juice may have even more fiber than raw tomatoes.

Most spaghetti and other pastas are made from refined grain flour, which has two-thirds of the fiber removed. To get all the natural fiber, choose whole wheat pastas, bulgar wheat and other whole grain products. For maximizing weight loss, eating foods high in fiber is even more essential.

Sugars (simple carbohydrates) come in many different forms, but the body utilizes them all in much the same way. Glucose, the body's primary fuel, is the dominant sugar in the blood. The body makes glucose from complex carbohydrates (starches), proteins and fats. We do not have to consume any sugar to have enough glucose. The liver breaks down the sugars we eat while a hormone, insulin, allows the cells to absorb the glucose and use it for energy. What isn't needed for immediate energy is stored in the liver and muscles as glycogen, or is converted to fat and stored, usually in places we wish it wasn't.

Sugar has been blamed for almost every health problem, from obesity to hyperactivity. While sugar may not be the culprit as claimed, there is some evidence that it may be responsible, at least in part, for some health problems. Sugar is not nearly as much of a problem for many people as eating too much fat. People gain weight when they consume more calories than they burn. Per gram, fat contains more than twice the calories of sugar (carbohydrates), so it is more likely that fat consumption will promote more weight gain than sugar consumption. Analysis of food intake of thin people showed that they eat more sugar (but fewer fats) than obese people. Cookies, cakes and many sweets are also often high sources of fats, and what is called a sweet tooth may really be a craving for fats. No direct link has been found between heart disease and sugar consumption. While people who have diabetes should be careful about the amount and type of sugar they eat, there is no evidence that sugar causes this disease. The most probable risk factor for non-insulin-dependent diabetes is obesity. For people eating a well-balanced diet and getting regular aerobic exercise, moderate sugar consumption is not usually a problem.

Hypoglycemia (low blood sugar) is relatively rare, although many people who suffer from fatigue, light-headedness, drowsiness and anxiety often blame their symptoms on this disorder. Blood sugar rises after we eat a meal. As the liver makes insulin to utilize sugars and carbohydrates, blood sugar levels may drop somewhat for an hour or two. Most people do not suffer any negative effect from this normal process. Studies of people with chronic fatigue syndrome show that it is not related to blood sugar fluctuations.

A common myth is that sugar will give extra energy if taken before exercising or competing. Taking sweets just before a workout may bring on fatigue more rapidly, as sugar triggers the body's production of insulin, further lowering blood sugar available for quick energy. Marathons and triathlons are exceptions; if the workout lasts more than two hours, performance may be increased with a high-energy snack during the event.

Studies prove that the belief some children behave in unacceptable ways after eating sugar is false. The same kids behave the same way without the sugar. Sweets are a pleasure food for most people. Many fruits are sought after mainly for their sweet taste, and are seldom eaten if not ripe, even though unripe fruit usually has equal nutritional value. While some people think sugar is addictive, there is no scientific evidence for this belief. Some people seem able to become "addicted" to almost anything, but this is more a reflection of their lack of self-control than of any physical or chemical dependence. While we can all live without eating refined sugars, the control of sweets can be a serious problem for some people.

Food labelers often hide sugars in their products by calling them other names. They also use more than one kind of sugar so that sugar will not have to be listed first, as the most common ingredient. In a list of ingredients, sugar can be called corn syrup, corn sweetener, dextrose, fructose, glucose, sorbitol, mannitol, barley malt, grape sweetener, sorghum, lactose, maltose and honey. For example, if two of these "hidden" sugars are listed as the third and fourth ingredients, it may be that sugar is actually the greatest ingredient in the product.

A number of delicious products have come on the market proudly proclaiming they are "Fat Free" and contain no refined sugars. Sweetened with fruit juices and concentrates, they are much more healthful than many traditional confections and may contain fiber, but they are still high in sugar. The result is high calories with less nutritional benefit than many natural foods. For those with less than perfect willpower, these products can become an irresistible temptation. Sweets often create a craving for more of the same, and can fill a person without providing the fiber and nutrients needed. If you have a weakness for sweets, be sure to limit your consumption to small amounts of these "healthy" products.

The pharmacy in your refrigerator will most likely amaze you. Almost all vegetables and fruits contain a combination of *phytochemicals,* compounds that help avoid cancer by preventing carcinogens from binding with DNA. Phytochemicals also increase the efficiency of the body's immune system. They can cause a form of a hormone, estrogen, to fragment into a harmless variant rather than the one that can lead to breast cancer. Broccoli is rich in these compounds. Tomatoes contain substances that prevent cancer-causing cell unions. Garlic and onions may not ward off vampires, but they do activate enzymes that protect against stomach cancer and help reduce cholesterol. Berries and citrus fruits are rich in flavonoids that prevent cells from joining with cancer-causing hormones. Soybeans, in their natural form or in tofu or miso, prevent some kinds of tumors from connecting to capillaries, preventing them from growing (but soy products are typically high in fat, so look for low-fat or "lite" tofu and other soy products). Hot peppers contain capsaicin, a substance known to keep toxins, like tobacco smoke, from binding with DNA, which can bring about lung cancer.

12

Fats

The role of dietary fat is one of the most commonly misunderstood areas of nutrition. In recent years a clear link has been established between the consumption of fat and heart disease, as well as many forms of cancer, diabetes and other health problems. We often hear it said that some kinds of fats are "better for you" than others. It would be more accurate to say that some kinds of fats are even more harmful than others. *Any* types of fats added to your diet are potentially harmful. What is most misunderstood is that, without adding any fat or oil, we get all the fat we need from a well-balanced diet of vegetables, whole grains, beans and legumes, and fruit.

Fats have many important functions. They store energy until it is needed and insulate the body with adipose cells that can expand like balloons. They also keep hair and skin healthy. Fats supply essential fatty acids (elements the body cannot make by itself) which help control blood pressure and other body functions through hormone-like compounds. Fats in food also give the feeling of being full for a longer time, since they slow down the process of digestion.

Americans consume more than 40 percent of their calories from fats. It's easier to get your calories from fats because ounce for ounce they contain more than twice as many calories as protein or carbohydrates. Even small amounts of oil have more calories than most people realize. A tablespoon of any kind of oil (13.5 grams) has over 120 calories. Many recipes call for a quarter of a cup of oil, butter, margarine or mayonnaise, adding nearly 1,000 calories.

Nutritional measures are usually listed in grams. There are 28⅓ grams in an ounce. A common paper clip weighs about one half of one gram (500 milligrams). A small avocado, after being peeled and pitted, will yield slightly more than an ounce (33 grams) of edible fruit. With 94 percent of its calories from fat, that small portion, less than 2½ tablespoons, has 280 calories.

Almost all health authorities agree that we should cut down on our intake of fats. Some of them would be happy if we reduced the amount by a quarter of the average American intake, to 30 percent of our calories. Others say it needs to be cut in half, to 20 percent. Drs. Ornish and McDougall, along with many others who have thoroughly studied this subject, have determined that we can get all our nutritional requirements for an active and productive life with just 10 percent of our calories from fat. Maintaining this 10 percent level is essential to reversing heart disease, and preventing and fighting some kinds of cancers, as well as benefiting the immune system. It also has a significant effect in reducing the effects of arthritis, allergies, diabetes and other cardiovascular-related illnesses.

Fats, also called *lipids,* are found in foods as triglycerides, so called because they have three fatty acids attached to a saturated, monounsaturated and polyunsaturated. Fats high in *saturated* fatty acids are commonly solid at room temperature. Butter and most animal fats are examples. These saturated fats (fully saturated with hydrogen atoms) raise cholesterol and are a primary contributor to heart disease. *Monounsaturated* fats (which can carry more hydrogen) and *polyunsaturated* fats (which are the least loaded with hydrogen atoms) are also called oils because they usually remain liquid at room temperature. There are claims that some unsaturated oils will help reduce cholesterol, but they actually have little beneficial effect. A balanced diet of vegetables, legumes, grains and fruits will lower cholesterol more quickly and safely and contain enough fats to meet our nutritional needs.

Table 12.1. Comparison of Fats

Rounded to nearest whole number (13.5 grams = one tablespoon)
Ranked in order of increasing danger for cholesterol and heart disease

Oil (13 grams)	Saturated grams	Monounsaturated grams	Polyunsaturated grams
Almond	1	10	2
Canola	1	8	4
Olive	2	10	1
Peanut	2	6	5
Corn	2	3	8
Cottonseed	4	2	7
Safflower	1	2	10
Sesame	2	5	6
Soybean	2	3	8
Sunflower	1	3	9
Margarine *	2	4	4
Lard	5	6	2
Butter	8	4	1

*Margarine has about 11 grams of fat per 13.5-gram tablespoon; the rest is water, flavors and fillers. Light margarines have more water, fillers and air, and may have fewer grams of fat per tablespoon.

This comparison chart shows different commonly used oils and some animal fats. All have the same fat content per gram, but the saturated portion varies greatly. An oil with fewer saturated fats is not "good" for you. All oils are 100 percent fat. Food can be sautéed in water, soy sauce, wine or balsamic vinegar, and although it will take a bit longer to cook at a reduced heat, the full flavor of most foods can be brought out without oils. Onion and garlic can be browned in a non-stick pan with a little water, and as they caramelize, they are just as sweet as when cooked in oil. Many spices can be roasted or broiled to bring out their flavor, either in a conventional oven or microwave. Most margarines are made from vegetable oils, water and sometimes a stabilizer or gelatin. Whipped margarines have air blended into them. To make these oils solid at room temperature, they are hydrogenated (by adding hydrogen atoms), a process that gives them nearly the same qualities as saturated fats. The body treats them as saturated fats, and they are as harmful as naturally saturated fats in raising blood cholesterol.

Fats are the most concentrated source of energy we can consume, providing more than twice the energy (calories) of sugar. Many people try to reduce by cutting down on sweets but continue to consume a high-fat diet. For weight control, sugar is only a small part of the problem. Sometimes the fat in foods isn't obvious. Those famous circular chocolate sandwich cookies with the white filling in the middle will surprise you. That filling is essentially vegetable shortening and sugar. Would you take a tablespoon of Crisco and mix it with a tablespoon of sugar and then eat it, or feed it to your kids? The only way to know what you're eating is to read labels carefully. (See chapter 20, "Reading Labels," for more information.)

The best way to cut down on fats is to avoid using them. It isn't necessary to give up all your favorite foods. Many pretzels are fat-free, and nearly fat-free potato and corn tortilla chips, baked instead of fried, are available. A single serving of a dozen regular fried tortilla chips can have from 6 to 14 grams of fat. A serving of corn chips that have been baked instead of fried, twice the size of the fried ones, has less than 1 gram of fat (from the corn itself). Baked chips will have nearly twice as many chips in a seven-ounce bag, since at least half the weight of fried chips is oil.

Cooking at home allows us to control fats, but when eating out it is much more difficult. Some restaurants will serve steamed vegetables and then cover them with butter. Others claim to add only a "little bit" of oil, but that small amount can bring the calories from fat to well over 50 percent. See chapter 19 on Eating Out and Traveling for survival tips and tricks.

Many adults feel they can cut back on fats, but worry about their children. Research findings and studies conducted in countries where fat is not commonly eaten show that after age two, children do not need the amounts of fat we usually give them. A reduction in fat for young children is one of the best insurance policies to prevent heart disease and some forms of cancer. Children who consume more fat than needed have higher cholesterol levels and more illnesses.

It isn't necessary to count calories or memorize the fat content of all the foods you eat. Cutting down on fat is easy. Avoid any food that has more than 3 grams of fat per serving. Know which foods are high in fat (avocados, nuts, seeds, olives and coconut are the most common) and learn to read labels. Find ways to avoid oil in cooking and in salad dressings. These few rules will keep you from making poor choices. You'll be eating close to 10 percent calories from fat, lowering your heart risk, gaining more energy, losing extra weight and improving your health.

There are many books listing foods and their fat content, but here is a small list of some common foods and their percentage of calories from fat (CFF). You may find a few surprises here:

Table 12.2. Percentage of Calories from Fat (CFF)

Animal Foods	%CFF	Plant Foods	%CFF
Spam	84	Tofu	49
Pork sausage	83	Mori-Nu lite tofu	28
Hot dogs	80	Mustard greens	13
Spareribs	80	Lettuce	12
Roast duck	76	Garbanzo beans	11
Salami	76	Mushrooms	8
Top loin steak	69	Cauliflower	7
Baked ham, lean	69	Cabbage	7
Tuna, oil pack	68	Eggplant	7
Fried chicken	65	Cucumber	6
Roast chicken	56	Apple	6
Anchovies	54	Papaya	4
Sea bass	53	Carrots	4
Mackerel, Pacific	49	Green peas	4
Salmon, red	49	Kidney beans	4
Beef stew	47	Onions	3
Roast turkey, leg	47	Potatoes	1

Fat shown on packages is by weight. Often packers will add water, causing the percentage to appear lower. Ham labeled "98 percent fat free" can have more than 50 percent of its calories from fat. "Extra lean" ground beef, labeled as "10 percent or less fat," usually has at least 49 percent of its calories from fat.

A number of products on the market claim to "burn" fat. Some have directions that instruct you to take the pills and do an hour of aerobic exercise. The fat is burned from the exercise, not the pill. Losing fat is most safely and permanently accomplished by eating wisely (lowering your fat intake) and exercising.

■ 13

Carbohydrates

Starches, sugars and some fiber that can be absorbed and used for energy are carbohydrates. For many years, many mistakenly believed that starches caused weight gain. As a result, many people tried to reduce their weight by reducing their intake of carbohydrates. Food scientists have since learned that we can maintain optimum health and fitness if we increase our carbohydrate intake to 75 or 80 percent of the calories we eat, and at the same time reduce fats and protein. A simple way to understand the principle behind a comparison of starches, fats and protein is to realize that all carbohydrates have four calories per gram, whether sugar or a starch. Fat has over twice that, nine calories per gram. An eight-ounce baked potato has 1 gram of fat and 25 grams of carbohydrates, totaling 110 calories. A four-ounce lean beef hamburger patty has 24 grams of fat and almost no carbohydrates, with a total of 350 calories. Rice, whole grains and pasta are examples of high carbohydrate foods.

The body converts dietary fat into body fat more efficiently than it converts carbohydrates into body fat. Studies show that when the body gets 100 extra calories from fat, only 3 calories are used to convert them, with 97 calories going to storage as fat, to be used later for energy. For every extra 100 carbohydrate calories you consume, about 23 will be burned up just in processing them. The other 77 will be stored as fat. When you eat carbohydrates, your chance of storing their calories as fat is 20 percent lower. Even better, since carbohydrates have only four calories a gram, while fat has nine, you can eat over twice the amount of carbohydrate-based foods than fat-based foods and still get fewer calories.

The body turns almost all carbohydrates into *glucose,* the primary fuel of the body and the dominant sugar in the blood.

Simple carbohydrates are sugars. It doesn't matter if they come from fruit, vegetables or honey; they all have about the same nutritional and caloric value. These are sometimes called "empty calories" because (with the exception of black strap molasses) they have little nutritional value. Dietary sugars are broken down into their simplest form, glucose and fructose, and are absorbed into the cells for energy.

Complex carbohydrates are glucose molecules usually combined with fiber, cellulose and starches. They provide more nutritional variety than simple carbohydrates and are a major source of dietary fiber, which is not found in animal products. Soluble fiber is an important factor in lowering blood cholesterol, but it has become an increasingly smaller part of the typical American diet, mostly due to the popularity of white flour, which has very little fiber. Whole wheat flour and other whole grains are rich in fiber and complex carbohydrates. Two slices of whole wheat bread have about 140 calories, while a soft drink has about 150. A soft drink is basically sugar (simple carbohydrates), while whole wheat bread is made from mostly complex carbohydrates, dietary fiber, and a variety of vitamins, minerals and essential amino acids. While some sugar is not harmful, we can get all of the sugars we need from fruits, vegetables and whole grains.

Many people believe carbohydrates are "fattening," but carbohydrates are not nearly as responsible for weight gain as fats are. Cakes, pies and baked sweets usually contain more fats than they do sugars. Pasta, rice and beans have about 20 grams of complex carbohydrates per half-cup, cooked, and not 1 gram of sugar. Potatoes, peas and corn have 12 grams of complex carbohydrates per half-cup, and only 3 grams of sugars (simple carbohydrates). Most vegetables are high in fiber, low in sugar, and almost all are rich in complex carbohydrates.

■ 14

Protein

P rotein deficiency is a terrible thing. You may have seen the effects in pictures of the bloated bellies of starving children. Ironically, in industrialized countries, more health problems are the result of an *excess* of protein in the diet. It is now well established that too much fat can be harmful to one's health, but many people still mistakenly believe that there's no such thing as too much protein. That can be a serious mistake.

About 20 percent of our body is made up of proteins. Bones, skin, muscles, cartilage, all enzymes and some hormones are basically protein, in tens of thousands of complex chains of amino acids. Through a process known as *protein turnover,* our body breaks down proteins, recycling most amino acids. Some new amino acids must be added, and the proteins we eat are needed for nearly all our internal processes to continue. While plants and bacteria can manufacture all 22 amino acids necessary for their existence, our bodies can only produce 13 of the 22. Because our bodies produce these 13 amino acids, they are not required in the foods we eat: these are called *nonessential amino acids.* The other nine amino acids that we need, the *essential amino acids,* must be supplied in our diet. All these can be obtained directly from plant foods (or indirectly from animals that have eaten plant foods). Contrary to what is often believed, it is *not* necessary to eat meat, fish or fowl to have all the essential amino acids in a balanced supply.

As the foods we eat are broken down into the various amino acids, the body's cells select what it needs to make its building blocks. Since there are nine amino acids that cannot be made within the body, it is important to eat foods that supply these. Combinations of vegetables, grains and fruits supply these essential nine amino acids, even if eaten at different meals several hours apart. For optimum health and growth, adults need only 10 to 15 percent of their calories from protein. Meats, eggs and dairy products contain up to 40 percent protein but not all of it is available because these are more difficult to digest. Most vegetables and grains are reasonably low in protein, almost all of it available through digestion. Some beans (and a few vegetables) are as high in protein as meats, and when eaten with grains and vegetables supply a healthful balance of complete protein, carbohydrates and fats.

The standard American diet is too high in animal proteins, leading to loss of calcium in the body. This can cause osteoporosis, a condition that makes bones brittle. Unfortunately, many people are told to drink milk and eat dairy foods to avoid or alleviate osteoporosis, but the high protein content in milk more than offsets the calcium it provides, so milk may actually lead to calcium loss. High levels of protein are also linked to kidney disease, resulting from the extra strain of filtering waste during protein breakdown. Animal protein and fats are linked to immune system deficiencies. To help your body prevent and fight disease, from flu to cancer, your immune system should be at its most efficient. Avoiding foods high in fat and cholesterol, as most animal foods are, and getting regular aerobic exercise is the best prescription for good health. Some weight training will also help prevent bone loss.

An old myth that continues to circulate is that more protein is needed to gain greater strength and athletic performance. It has been repeatedly scientifically demonstrated that this is not true. Excess protein is either excreted or, more commonly, converted to fat. Whether this extra protein is consumed in foods or in supplements, the body treats it in the same way.

Claims that one vitamin or mineral supplement has amino acids and is more readily absorbed than others is a reflection on how little the public knows about the body's use of proteins. For persons wanting to *gain* weight, these supplements are probably beneficial, but that gain will be primarily fat, not muscle, unless a rigorous exercise program is followed. Exercise is what builds muscles. Supplements and energy foods are never directly turned into muscle. Many other claims have been made for various amino acids, from curing diseases to preventing insomnia. There is no scientific evidence that over-the-counter amino acid supplements cure anything. However, large doses of some have been linked to the development of some health problems, and the FDA has tried to stop sales of megadoses of amino acids.

The average American consumes over 100 grams of protein a day, more than three times the amount needed for optimum health and nutrition. To reverse heart disease, you should limit your intake of protein to between 10 and 15 percent of calories. By eating a variety of vegetables, whole grains, legumes (beans, lentils, peas) and fruit, you'll get all the protein you need.

15

Calcium

One of the most common nutritional myths is that you must eat dairy products to get enough calcium. Milk holds a special place in American culture, next to apple pie and Mother. The dairy industry has convinced most of us that we can't live without its products, but there is ample evidence that we can live longer, feel better and have as much strength without milk, cheese, yogurt and all other dairy products.

Most of the calcium in the body is in our bones, with a small amount in the bloodstream to help regulate the heartbeat, transmission of nerve impulses and muscle contraction. The amount of calcium in the blood is controlled by hormones. Calcium is continuously lost through body waste and sweat, and is replaced with calcium from the bones. As a process of normal tissue growth, the body constantly breaks down bone material and rebuilds it, using calcium from foods for replacement.

Keeping bones strong depends more on preventing calcium loss than on increasing calcium intake. In nations with high rates of osteoporosis, protein intake is generally more than twice the U.S. Recommended Daily Allowance. Diets high in protein, especially animal protein, cause calcium to be lost through the urine. Meats are high in a particular kind of protein building block, called sulfur-containing amino acids, that increases calcium loss. Studies show that vegetarians are less than half as likely to suffer osteoporosis than meat eaters are. Caffeine and sodium also increase the rate of calcium loss through urine. Alcohol inhibits calcium absorption and may also be toxic to bone. We can benefit from boron, found in fruits, vegetables and beans, since it appears to help stop the loss of calcium. Vitamin D, copper, zinc and weight training exercise also may increase bone mass and help prevent osteoporosis.

The need for calcium varies at different ages. For the first 35 years, our bodies lose less calcium than we consume. After 45, our bodies gradually lose more calcium than we take in. The rate of calcium loss depends on how much and what kind of protein we consume. A negative calcium balance can result in osteoporosis.

The body regulates how much calcium it absorbs, usually between 30 and 70 percent for a normal diet. If a person eats more calcium, the body just doesn't absorb it. This is a reason why high doses of calcium supplements may not prevent bone loss.

Milk is *not* the ideal way to get your daily supply of calcium. Milk (except skim) is high in saturated fat. It also contains high amounts of calcium-blocking protein. In addition, antibiotics fed to cows are passed on in about one-third of the milk sold in America. Also, bovine growth hormone is now allowed to be given to dairy cows to increase their milk supply. This hormone, usually combined with greater amounts of antibiotics, has not been subjected to long-term human testing.

Although they often don't realize it, most people (about 75 percent of the U.S. population) have an allergy to cow's milk, called lactose intolerance. As infants, our bodies make an enzyme called *lactase,* allowing us to metabolize milk sugars (lactose). After childhood, most people no longer make this enzyme. As a result, their bodies see the lactose in dairy products as an alien invader, and trigger allergic reactions. Human breast milk provides all the calcium a child needs and has only 6 percent of calories from protein, far less than the 22 percent in cow's milk, which is the amount needed for a *calf* to grow quickly. Dark green leafy vegetables are a much better source of calcium than milk, and they have almost no fat and much lower amounts of protein. Some plant sources of calcium are shown in appendix F.

16

Iron

One of the common beliefs about a vegetarian diet is that it doesn't supply enough iron. Vegetarians do not have a higher incidence of iron deficiency than meat eaters. While animal proteins and dairy products do have iron, some plant foods are even richer. Iron deficiency anemia is most commonly found in young women and children who are currently eating red meat, fowl and fish.

Iron is a central part of hemoglobin, carrying oxygen in the blood. It is found in food in two forms. The first type, about 40 percent of the iron in meat, poultry and fish, is well absorbed. The other type, 100 percent of the iron in plant foods and 60 percent of the iron in animal tissue, is somewhat less well absorbed, when isolated.

Because vegetarians eat the form of iron that is not as well absorbed, it is often believed that they will develop iron deficiency anemia, but this is not the case. Iron absorption is reduced by some foods. Tannin in tea binds iron in the intestines, decreasing its absorption. Drinking tea between meals or using herbal teas would allow better iron absorption than taking tea with meals. This absorption factor causes some confusion, but it is not an important issue for those eating a well-balanced vegetarian diet.

Most vegetarian diets are high in ascorbic acid (vitamin C), which increases iron absorption up to six times, making the absorption of plant-based iron as good as or better than animal-based iron. Many vegetables, such as broccoli and bok choy, are high in iron and in vitamin C, so that the iron in these foods is well absorbed. Beans and tomato sauce or stir-fried tofu and broccoli, common vegetarian combinations, allow generous levels of iron absorption. The iron in plant foods is superior to that derived from animal foods when the amount of iron per calorie is considered. Just 100 calories of spinach has as much iron as 340 calories of sirloin steak.

Instead of worrying about not getting enough iron, people with a high heart risk factor should make sure they're not getting too much. Clinical studies have shown that high iron levels may be related to heart disease. Men who take a multivitamin daily should be sure that iron is not one of the minerals included. The RDA for iron is 15 milligrams per day for an adult woman. Men and post-menopausal women only need 10 milligrams daily. The iron content of some common foods is given in appendix E.

17

Water

Because it has no calories, you might not think water is an essential element in nutrition and the reduction of heart attack risk, but it is a highly important aspect of health. Among its many functions, water keeps our kidneys functioning efficiently. When the kidneys cannot do their job properly, the liver must take on some of that task. If this happens, it cannot metabolize fat into energy as well. Water also aids in digestion, carries nutrients, aids in building tissue, transports waste from the body and helps maintain the body's normal temperature.

About 60 percent of a person's weight is made up of water. A fluid loss of as little as 2 percent of body weight can affect physical performance. A 5 percent loss can cause stomach and muscle cramps. Heat stroke, which can be fatal, often occurs at 7 to 10 percent fluid loss. Although there are large amounts of water in vegetables and fruit, which is helpful to vegetarians, anyone who consumes high levels of fiber should be sure to consume sufficient water.

Contrary to what many people think, a good way to combat excess fluid retention is to drink water. When the body doesn't get enough water, it conserves all the moisture it can. The extracellular spaces it is stored in (swollen feet, hands and legs) hoard the water until the threat of dehydration is no longer sensed. The best way to tell your body to release the stored fluids is to give it water. Salt can cause higher water retention, requiring extra water to dilute it. Lowering salt intake is easy to do, and extra amounts of water will flush the sodium from the system.

Thirst is not always a good indication of the need for water. In many people, the sensation of thirst doesn't occur until the body is already dangerously dehydrated. The best way to assure a proper fluid balance for an average size person is to drink at least six to eight 8-ounce glasses of water a day. Heavier people need to drink even more water. A half-hour heavy workout can produce as much as three quarts of sweat, a 4 percent fluid loss for a 150-pound person. That loss needs to be replaced. Beyond the basic six to eight glasses of water a day, for each 100 pounds of body weight, an additional 8-ounce cup of water should be taken for each hour of light exercise, 14 ounces (1½ cups) for moderate exercise and 20 ounces (2½ cups) of water for each hour of strenuous activity.

Plain cool (not iced) water is the best way to replace fluid loss. Fruit juice, mixed half and half with water, or sports drinks with not more than 10 percent carbohydrate concentration are also good. High-carbohydrate sports drinks (more than 24 grams of carbohydrate per eight ounces) are not advised. Sodas, undiluted fruit juices and high-carbohydrate drinks actually slow down water absorption and do not allow immediate fluid replacement.

In exercise lasting up to 1½ hours, taking small sips of water or low-carbohydrate sports drinks is often helpful, but it is better to avoid drinking large amounts while exercising. For marathons and long exercise sessions, larger quantities of fluids are needed. For these longer events, a good test is to weigh yourself before and after. For each pound of weight loss, you should drink 16 ounces (two cups) of water.

Some drinks, such as coffee and tea, can increase fluid loss because they have a diuretic effect. Alcohol is a stronger diuretic; the body needs eight ounces of water to replace the loss from just one ounce of pure alcohol. Hot weather and low humidity can add to the dehydration effect. Almost all foods contain water, but they also may contain carbohydrates, protein and fiber, which increase the need for water. Vegetables range from 70 to 90 percent water and can be used as a part of the six to eight cups of water needed daily.

If you decide to suddenly increase your water intake, you may find that it will take two or three weeks for your system to become accustomed to the change. You'll likely make more frequent trips to the bathroom for a week or two, but your bladder will gradually become used to handling the increased flow, and your routine will soon return to normal.

Water is not a substitute for foods, but it can help you avoid the temptation of high-calorie or high-fat offerings, especially when you're away from home. A large glass of water just before you are tempted may help you control your craving.

18

Other Health Benefits

Changing to a low-fat vegetarian diet and practicing regular aerobic exercise are vital to reversing heart disease, but the benefits don't stop there. Many other common health problems are more closely related to diet and fitness than was previously believed. While you're lowering your heart attack risk, you are extending the length and quality of your life in other ways.

Cancers are not all alike, and the reasons we get some types of cancer are not fully understood. Much has been learned in recent years about how cancer cells grow and how the body tries to fight them. As the body of information grows, diet is being recognized as a major factor affecting the immune system and the way the body deals with cancer. Some types of cancer are linked to diet, including breast, prostate, intestinal, colon and some skin cancers. In countries with low fat and high fiber consumption, such cancers are rare. Not only does low fat and high fiber consumption help prevent heart disease; they are important in how well the body works to prevent free radicals from damaging cells, believed to be the origin of many cancers. Foods containing beta-carotene and vitamin C are rich in antioxidants that defend against free radicals. Many green, leafy vegetables have cancer-fighting components. Studies also show that these lifestyle changes have brought about improvement in people already diagnosed with some kinds of cancer.

Diabetes used to be thought of as a disease of the obese. While being overweight increases the risk, it is not the only factor. The major type (95 percent) of diabetes is called *adult-onset* or *non-insulin-dependent diabetes.* Insulin injections are not always required for control of adult-onset diabetes. A rarer form of diabetes, *childhood-onset,* occurs when there isn't enough insulin in the body, and injections or oral medications are usually required. Both types are related to high levels of blood sugar. In adult-onset diabetes, the body has insulin, but it isn't as efficient in helping cells accept sugar for energy conversion.

The pancreas makes the insulin needed to balance the sugar in the blood. If the cells can't get energy from blood sugars, they get it from body fats, but this can cause chemical imbalances that affect metabolism and many other functions. The effects of diabetes make it difficult for the body to recover from injury and minor infections, and can result in the amputation of an arm or leg, loss of eyesight or even death. Diabetics are more susceptible to strokes, cancer, high blood pressure, heart attacks, kidney failure, gout, blindness and gangrene.

The lifestyle recommendations made here for lowering heart disease risk apply to preventing and fighting diabetes. The intake of simple carbohydrates (sugar) must be carefully controlled, but some physicians are not aware that an increased intake of complex carbohydrates can be beneficial in treating diabetes, perhaps because they group all carbohydrates together. Following this book's nutrition and exercise suggestions and giving more attention to limiting fruits and other simple carbohydrates usually has a positive effect in controlling diabetes, often allowing people to lower or discontinue medication. (*A caution for insulin users:* when beginning these lifestyle changes, improvements can occur so rapidly that it is advisable to test yourself at least four times a day and to adjust your dosage accordingly.)

Allergies often are more related to what we eat than other factors we are led to believe are their origin. People suffering from a runny nose and stuffed head often blame these symptoms on pollen or other airborne pollutants. Many of these symptoms go away after changing to a very low-fat vegetarian diet. One of the most common food allergies is to dairy proteins and lactose (a sugar found in milk). As many as 95 percent of some ethnic groups have lactose intolerance, yet most consume milk, cheese or yogurt daily. A common benefit reported by many *Healing Heart* support group participants is relief from allergies they had suffered for years.

Arthritis and diet are related, but it seems not all physicians are aware of this link. Recent research studies have established a clear relationship between diet and arthritis. Ironically, gout is much like arthritis, and doctors often tell gout patients that diet is an important part of getting relief. If you have arthritis, write down the type and the frequency of pain (or restriction of movement) for a few days before you start the recommended lifestyle changes, then see if these remain a few weeks later. One *Healing Heart* group member who came to reduce high cholesterol wrote her name on the chalkboard during the fifth week, announcing with considerable emotion that she was now able use her hands to write and do things she hadn't been able to do for over 15 years. She told the group that regardless of her cholesterol, she would continue her new eating habits for the rest of her life, if only for the arthritis relief.

Osteoporosis is a loss of bone mass that affects nearly 20 million people in the U.S. alone. As the bone loses minerals, especially calcium, it becomes weak and brittle. Over a million bone fractures each year are blamed on osteoporosis. When this condition progresses far enough, the weight of the rest of the body alone can cause bones to break apart without any other force or injury. Although osteoporosis is considered a hazard of getting older, it does not have to be part of the aging process. Women from Western industrialized countries are particularly susceptible to osteoporosis, since they consume high amounts of dairy products and other proteins. In women, the effects begin after age 40 and become much greater after menopause. Estrogen therapy can slow osteoporosis down, but not reverse it. Men also can have osteoporosis, but it is usually much less severe and doesn't become apparent until the mid-1970s. Only proper diet and weight-bearing exercise can stop osteoporosis and actually increase bone mass as we get older.

Skin problems, such as acne, are diet-related in most people. Dr. Terry Shintani, a physician with an advanced degree in nutrition, advises a low-fat vegetarian diet. He announced on his radio program that most of the people with acne who started this diet had clearer skin in weeks. The typical diet of teenagers, burgers and fries, pizza and other high-fat fast foods, aggravates their skin condition. Applying expensive ointments over irritated skin can help hide blemishes and reduce infection, but healthier nutrition will often clear skin more quickly and permanently.

Constipation is a common complaint, clearly evident from the large variety of laxatives on sale at any drugstore. When elimination is difficult or infrequent, a number of problems can occur. The exertion can cause varicose veins, hemorrhoids, bowel and colon irritation and hernias. One of the most common places where people suffer strokes is in the bathroom, straining against constipation. No animal products contain dietary fiber, which is needed to assure the easy passage of waste. Adopting the dietary recommendations in this book should relieve constipation. Eating the recommended servings of vegetables, whole grains, fresh fruit, beans and other legumes, and drinking plenty of water, will usually eliminate constipation and end the need to take fiber supplements or laxatives.

Looking at the many health benefits of the lifestyle changes recommended here, it may sound as though these changes will cure just about anything. Obviously they won't, but there are more than enough advantages in this lifestyle to give almost anyone good reasons to start the program. This is not magic. The guidelines are based on published scientific studies accepted after careful review. The recommended lifestyle can not only result in reversal of coronary artery disease and reduced heart risk factors, but can help your entire body function at its most efficient level, making a difference in health, energy and longevity.

19

Eating Out and Traveling

Preparing meals at home may not be as convenient as eating out or ordering take-out foods, but when you make things yourself you can keep the amount of fat, sugar and sodium to acceptable limits. When going to restaurants, parties, potlucks and barbecues, it becomes a challenge to avoid fats and animal proteins. There are a variety of ways in which you can eat enough and still enjoy the occasion.

Restaurants that offer vegetarian and low-fat friendly foods are increasing, and many will go out of their way to give you a low-fat meal that is as delicious as their regular menu fare. The American Restaurant Association has informed its members that about 7 percent of the population, or about one in every 14 persons, requests vegetarian food. They urge their members to offer more vegetarian items. Unfortunately, vegetarian doesn't necessarily mean low fat. Vegetables may arrive covered in butter, margarine or oils. Salad dressings are mostly fat and many baked goods are high in oils.

Steamed vegetables are available in many restaurants. Baked potato is frequently offered, as are rice and pasta. A plate of vegetables and a potato or rice is filling and nutritious, especially if served with an oil-free spaghetti sauce or salsa. Salad bars are a good source, if you avoid the cheeses and dressings. I bring a small plastic jar of my own favorite non-fat salad dressing with me when I eat out, and I've never had a problem from anyone about this. Soft rolls and breads may have a little oil, but with the other items you're eating, the meal should still be less than 10 percent calories from fat. When whole wheat bread isn't available, French bread, which is usually made without oil, is the best choice (but without butter or margarine). If the dinner isn't too formal, I often make up a veggie sandwich, adding some non-fat salad dressing on the bread. Ketchup is a non-fat flavor enhancer, but mustard is a high-fat food, though small quantities are not a problem.

In the U.S. and Canada, most larger communities have ethnic restaurants. Vietnamese, Thai, Indian and other Asian restaurants often feature vegetarian dishes, but you should make it clear that you do not want oil or fat. Coconut milk is a common ingredient in many Southeast Asian dishes, so order with care. Chinese restaurants are found in even small communities, but their vegetarian dishes are often made with oil and chicken stock, and can be high in MSG. A personal request to the owner or manager will often get you low-fat and meatless versions of many menu items. I usually don't ask the waiter, since the cook may not care what he requests, but when the boss says low-fat, it is more likely to come that way. Europe and South America have fewer vegetarian resources, but asking around will almost always reveal at least one place to eat safely. The Vegetarian Resource Group (see Recommended Resources for address) and an Internet source has a list of restaurants in all areas of the world.

Calling the restaurant in advance can make the difference between a risky evening and a rewarding one. Explain that you must eat a "*no*-fat vegetarian" diet for health reasons. To some people "*low*-fat" might mean a meal with more fat than you'd want to eat in a week. The mention of heart disease usually promotes cooperation, since almost everyone knows someone who has it.

Many national restaurant chains offer low-fat choices. Veggieburgers are becoming more common. Gardenburgers (a brand of vegetarian patties made of oats and vegetables) are now available in more than 5,000 restaurants in the Los Angeles area alone. National restaurant chains may vary their menu from one location to another. The information that follows is subject to change, but reflects the trend of some restaurant chains to offer more vegetarian and low-fat choices. Some national chains change their menu from time to time, so check your local outlet's current offerings.

Fried Squid—No Squid

Before I started on this program, one of my favorite meals was a dish of fried squid, mostly fresh stir-fried vegetables and a tangy, spicy sauce served at a local Korean restaurant. I was sad to learn that the same size portion of squid has five times the cholesterol of steak, and it looked like I'd never get to eat my favorite dish again. When I asked for the fried squid dish, but without the squid, I explained that it was for my heart condition and I'd eat vegetarian or nothing. The owner agreed, but said she'd have to charge extra to leave out the squid. Although that sounded strange, I agreed. Then I told her that I wanted it cooked without oil. She shook her head and said that was impossible. So with great authority I told her that with the squid it needed oil, but without the fish, it could be prepared without any oil. She looked at me as if I were crazy, but made it my way. It was just as delicious as it had been in the past (in fact, with the spicy sauce, I'm not sure I ever tasted the squid), and I could eat it as often as I liked. Now she adds lots of extra vegetables and charges me the same as the original squid dish. Always ask for what you want, and take the time to explain why.

TGI Friday's restaurants usually have a light menu with at least two vegan (strictly vegetarian with no eggs or dairy) options, the vegetable baguette (ordered without cheese) and the Gardenburger. Santa Fe Chicken, which is a sliced breast of chicken or tuna over a bowl of mixed steamed vegetables, with a vinaigrette sauce on the side, can be ordered without the meat and with a baked potato. They also serve baked potatoes with steamed vegetables in them. The Thai chicken salad, ordered without the chicken, is mostly salad greens, oriental vegetables, Chinese noodles and mandarin orange slices in a spicy peanut dressing. The noodles and peanuts are high-fat, but they are a very small part, so the meal is within acceptable limits.

In an emergency, most Burger Kings offer a Veggie Whopper. This is a Whopper sandwich without the meat or cheese. Ask for extra lettuce and tomato instead of the meat, and tell them to hold the mayonnaise. The price is the same as their regular Whopper. At one time, Burger King test-marketed a true low-fat veggie burger, had a surprisingly large number of sales, but then announced they would not offer it nationally. Ask the manager when they will offer it again, as they may bow to customer demand.

Taco Bell can make up a burrito with refried beans (which have a small amount of vegetable oil) and salsa. They also have a salad, but it is not very large or varied. Avoid the taco salad, which was analyzed to have 61 grams of fat even without the 50-percent fat taco shell. Their "lite" offerings have much less fat, but most still have 5 grams of fat or more.

Subway sandwich shops offer a veggie combination on a

whole wheat roll. It is made of the normal garnish that goes on their other sandwiches—lettuce, tomato, pickles, peppers, bean sprouts and cheese. Ask them to hold the cheese, olives and mayonnaise and you'll have a filling lunch. Subway shops' menus may vary, and some franchises offer fat-free veggie burgers. If your local Subway doesn't, enough requests may get them added to the menu.

Vegetarians across the U.S. report that Denny's does not appear to cater to persons seeking low-fat vegetarian food. They have discontinued their veggie sandwich and the menu offers little else that is within the guidelines recommended here.

Many local restaurants and regional chains offer excellent low-fat vegetarian choices. If you find one, it is a good idea to thank the manager. Telling those in charge that their offerings are appreciated helps keep these items on the menu and encourages them to add more.

At dinner parties it is both courteous and wise to call the hosts and explain your dietary restrictions. Usually just explaining that you'd appreciate no meat, fish or fowl for yourself and that you can simply double up on vegetables and starches will get you a fine meal without embarrassing yourself or the hosts by asking for special treatment at the time the meal is served.

At potlucks I bring a dish to share and also bring enough to feed myself in a separate container. If the other choices allow me to eat what is offered, I can take my emergency meal home. At a barbecue or other buffet where there may not be much for me to choose from, I eat a full meal before leaving, and then I snack on a salad, vegetables or bread if there is any. If I have to be there for a while before I can eat, I ask the hosts if it is okay to bring special diet food with me. Many hosts offer to make something special for me, but I always decline, saying that I'm happy to bring my own.

Traveling, especially when the meals are prepared in

advance, can be risky. I always bring plenty of low-fat snacks with me when flying, such as whole wheat bagels, pretzels (I scrape off the salt) and fruit. Almost all airlines offer special meals, vegetarian, low-fat, non-dairy, kosher and others. It is important to order these meals well in advance, when making reservations, and to confirm the request a day or two before departing. That doesn't mean you'll get the meal, though. When the meal service starts, the cabin attendants may ask who gets the vegetarian meal. If someone who either forgot to order one or decides that it sounds good raises a hand, your pre-ordered meal may go to someone else. Before departure, it is helpful to tell the cabin attendant responsible for your area that you ordered a special meal. It's also a good idea to give a gentle reminder just before the meals are served. If you find your meal has been served to someone else or not even loaded on the airplane, ask for a fruit plate and any extra veggies and get your emergency rations ready.

When taking long car trips, sandwiches can be made in advance, salads made along the way, and other foods stored in a cooler. If you're traveling with kids who want fast-food stops, bring your own food with you to eat while the kids have theirs.

■ 20

Reading Labels

Proper nutrition doesn't occur accidentally. Careful reading of food labels is the best way to find out whether packaged foods will decrease or increase your risk of heart attack. In 1994 a new food-labeling law became effective in the U.S. This new label has the words *Nutrition Facts* at the top. While the new law has some weaknesses, it is more informative than the prior one. Understanding how to read food labels is an important step toward getting the right balance of foods.

As fat becomes more commonly recognized as a source of health problems, many producers are making claims that their products are low-fat or fat-free. Often this is untrue. The labeling laws make this deception possible by using a small serving size and allowing grams of fat to be rounded off, so .49 grams of fat can be called zero. They realize that most consumers don't read or understand the labels. One margarine substitute has the words *fat free* in large letters on the

Figure 20.1. Nutrition Label

Nutrition Facts

Serving Size 1 oz. (22 chips)
Servings per Container 7

Amount per Serving

Calories 110
Calories from Fat 15

% Daily Value

Total Fat 1.5 g   2%

Saturated Fat 0 g   0%

Cholesterol 0 g   0%

Sodium 160 mg

Total Carbohydrate 34 g 8%

Dietary Fiber 3 g

Sugars less than 1 g

Protein 3 g

Vitamin A 2% • Vitamin C 8%
Calcium 10% • Iron 6%

Calories per gram
Fat 9 Carbohydrate 4 Protein 4

Current labels require serving sizes be more reasonable. In the past, the size was unrealistically small. Rules still let fat under .5 g show as zero.

Note the total calories per serving. We often eat more than one small serving.

Total fat is usually rounded off. Total fat times 9 gives the calories from fat. The total fat here is actually 1.7 g.

Avoid foods over 3 g **fat** per serving.

Saturated fat is most harmful type. If this number is high, avoid it.

Cholesterol is found only in animal products. Try to avoid *any* amount.

Limit **sodium** to 1000-2000 mg/day.

Complex carbohydrates are the best foods. 75% of calories should be these.

The higher the **fiber**, the better.

Sugars are simple carbohydrates. Limit them to a small percentage.

Keep **protein** below 15% of calories.

(See chapter for explanation)

The Daily Values shown are for the Standard American Diet (SAD) which is not heart healthy. The percentages at the right of the label and the list of daily values are not for those attempting to reduce their risk of heart disease. They can be safely ignored.

package, but reading the nutrition facts reveals that each serving has five calories, with five calories from fat. That means the product is just about 100 percent fat. Claims of being "97 percent fat free" are also misleading, since this is usually based on the weight of the product, not the calories from fat.

Don't worry about counting calories; you can eat all you want of low-fat foods. The *percent of calories from fat* is the number you need to know. It can be calculated by dividing the calories from fat by the total calories. In the following example, the calories from fat are 15 and the total calories are 110.

$$15 \div 110 = 0.136 \ (13.6\%)$$

In the labeling law, words sometimes don't mean what they usually do. Under pressure from food manufacturers who want to be able to make healthful claims, the FDA has approved some artificial definitions for terms. Here are their meanings on the label and what they mean to you. Claims of "Low Fat" and "Lite" may not be valid for persons attempting to lower their heart disease risk factor. Always read the Nutritional Facts portion of the label.

Table 20.1. Nutritional Claims

To Make a Claim About	FDA Says It Must Be	Health Meaning
Heart disease, fats	"low" in fat and cholesterol	"low" in fat and cholesterol is not defined in numbers; it can mean anything
Blood pressure, sodium specific	"low" in sodium	"low" in sodium is not an amount; sodium sensitive persons should use care

| Heart disease and fruits, vegetables and grain products | "low" in fat and cholesterol and contain at least 0.6 grams soluble fiber, without additions | some plant foods are higher in fat than others (avocados, olives, nuts, seeds, some beans); a few are high in saturated fats (coconuts, palm products); but no plant foods contain cholesterol |

Claims may mean the opposite of the nutritional truth:

Table 20.2. FDA Nutritional Claims

Claim	FDA Meaning (per serving)	Health Meaning
Fat free	less than 0.5 gram of fat	may be high in fat, if many servings used
Low fat	3 grams or less of fat	3 grams is *high* fat for heart health
Lean	less than 10 grams of total fat 4 grams of saturated fat and 95 milligrams of cholesterol	an artery clogging food to be avoided; 95 milligrams is a 3-week supply for those trying to reverse heart disease risks
Light (Lite)	30% fewer calories *or* half the fat and half the sodium of the regular version of the same food	doesn't mean it is low fat or low sodium, just that it has less than the item it is being compared with; could still be very high in fat and sodium
Cholesterol free	less than 2 milligrams of cholesterol and less than 2 grams of saturated fat	a good guide to cholesterol, but check the saturated fat: 2 grams is too much

Source: Food and Drug Administration, Washington, D.C.   FDA 93-2260

■ 21

Exercise

here are many different kinds of exercise, but the most important type for reversing heart disease is *aerobic* exercise. Lifting weights, isometrics, golf, tennis and even handball or racquetball, for all the sweat they produce, are not aerobic. Aerobic exercises require repeated regular movement of major muscle groups to bring the heartbeat up to a pre-determined level and keep it there continually for a specific period of time.

With aerobic exercise, different people can do much different levels of work and still be getting the same aerobic benefit. An overweight, out-of-shape person walking at 3.5 miles an hour may have a heart rate of 125 or more, but a thinner, more fit person may have to run at 6 miles an hour or faster to get to that same level. Age is also an important factor in determining what heart rate is best to provide maximum benefit without causing problems.

As you exercise, you'll need to gradually do more work

to keep your heart rate at the level you want. That means since your heart is better able to meet the demand that the exercise requires, it's working more efficiently. What used to be a real effort becomes easier to achieve. To gain the same benefits you'll gradually have to walk a little faster, or climb a slightly steeper hill, or maybe bike in a higher gear. As you become more fit, you'll find that your resting pulse will lower. Mine went from 72 beats per minute to 51 in just six months. Instead of having to work to push blood through the arteries 72 times every minute, it now has to do that only 51 times a minute. If I were resting all the time, that's over 30,000 muscle contractions a day it no longer has to make. When I'm active, it is saving my heart even more energy. Persons who are very much out of shape may start out with a resting pulse rate as high as 90 or more, but as exercise brings about better cardiovascular fitness, this will soon lower. If your resting pulse is above 85, you should consult your physician before starting any exercises. Some heart conditions can be made worse by going beyond a reasonable target heart rate. It is always best to start slowly and gradually build up to no more than 70 percent of maximum heart rate (MHR). You should check with your physician if you plan to go higher than 70 percent of your MHR.

To determine your maximum heart rate, subtract your age from 220. If you're in reasonably good health and not already exercising, start near to 45 percent of your MHR. In the past it was believed that all 40 minutes had to be at one time, but two 20-minute sessions, or even three 15-minute sessions will give you the aerobic workout you need. (*Caution:* Some calcium and beta blocker medications artificially lower heart rate; persons on blockers should not use this formula and should consult their physician for a target heart rate.)

At the same time that the heart muscles are becoming better able to do their job, the arteries that feed them are becoming better able to supply blood to those muscles. Exercise, in combination with proper diet, can actually open up these clogged arteries. If you've ever had a muscle cramp, you remember the pain your body uses to signal you to change your demand on that muscle group. Most often the cramp is due to an insufficient supply of blood to that muscle, usually because it was overtaxed or not ordinarily used in that particular way. As you build up your muscles, the blood vessels that supply them with fuel become better able to meet the increased demand. Your heart is muscle and it can be strengthened in the same manner as other muscles.

The Example of Lee

Let's take Lee, for example. At age 40, Lee's MHR would be 180 (220 minus 40 =180). Forty minutes a day between 45 percent to 70 percent of MHR is all that is needed to give Lee's heart and lungs the exercise they need. Using this example of an MHR of 180, Lee would start with a heart rate of 81 (180 times .45 = 81). Lee should try to keep his heart rate at 81 beats per minute for as much of the time as possible while walking or exercising. Instead of counting out a whole minute, it's easier to divide by 6 and count the pulse for 10 seconds (81 divided by 6 = 13.5). Counting the pulse for 10 seconds, there should be 13 or 14 beats. As exercise becomes easier, Lee would gradually move the target percentage up, first to 50% (15 beats in 10 seconds, or 90 beats a minute) and then, in small steps, all the way up to 21 beats in 10 seconds, or 125 beats a minute, to 70% of the MHR.

Walking is one of the best exercises for your heart. If you've recently had surgery or have angina, you may want to start slowly, with a brief stroll, and gradually increase to a brisk 45-minute walk. It helps to have a watch that will let you count the time you've taken to walk a particular route. If it's a short walk, you can do it several times a day, trying to shave a few seconds off your previous best time. Don't overdo it by trying too hard; you have a lifetime to get your heart in shape.

You can count the steps per minute to see how fast you are walking. Once you have a route to walk, measure the distance. When you know the time and distance, you'll be able to calculate your speed in miles per hour. Here's a rough guide to the number of steps per minute for various walking speeds and the number of calories you might burn while walking on a level surface on a 70° day:

Table 21.1. Calories Burned Walking

Steps per minute	Miles per hour	Calories per minute*	Calories per hour*
105	3.0	4	240
120	3.5	5	300
140	4.0	6	360
160	4.5	7	430
175	5.0	8	520

*Actual calories per minute burned depends on body weight, height and other factors. These numbers are for a 120-pound person. Heavier persons burn more calories. See the chart in the Appendix B for more information.

Another way to keep your speed is to listen to a tape that has a steady number of beats per second. A company called SportsMusic has a series of tapes at different exercise levels for walking, biking, treadmills and other machines, with tapes ranging from Dixieland to pop, showtunes to classical. Their address and toll-free phone are listed in the Recommended Resources section.

To get the best workout from walking, pump your arms (for increased cardiovascular effect), breathe deeply and use good posture, with your shoulders slightly back and your bottom tucked in. Walk on even surfaces, but do some stepping up and down on curbs and add some hills to vary your workout. Walking has the least possibility of injury of any of the popular exercises. Carrying weights while walking is not advised, and does not burn as many extra calories as walking an extra minute or two.

The aerobic benefit from other exercises compared with walking at 3½ miles per hour is shown below. For example, each mile of swimming is roughly the equivalent of three miles of walking.

Table 21.2. Aerobic Benefit of Exercise

Biking	0.5-1.5	Swimming	3.0
Running	1.5-3.0	Hiking (5% grade)	2.0
Aerobic dancing	3.5	Exerstriding	1.5
Rollerblading	0.5-1.0	Golfing (9 holes)	0.5-1.0

An excellent alternative to the usual exercise workout is Tai Chi Chuan. A series of stretching and balancing poses smoothly blended into one continuous and graceful movement, Tai Chi is one of Asia's most popular exercise forms. It is gentle enough that some people have been able to continue practicing it daily for over 90 years. While it is technically possible to learn Tai Chi from a book, the best way is to take a class. Some park and recreation districts and adult education services offer Tai Chi lessons.

Hatha yoga is another exercise form that is gaining much popularity. This form of yoga is a series of poses, called *asanas,* that help a person relax, stretch and tone muscle groups, and gain better balance. Iyengar is a style of hatha yoga a bit more physically demanding than some other forms, and allows a number of aids, such as belts and blocks, to make it easier for beginners to work into the more difficult poses. While hatha yoga has often been confused with Eastern religious practice, it does not need to conflict with any belief system or religion. Taken simply as an exercise form, it provides few aerobic benefits but adds many stretching and toning benefits to traditional aerobic exercise. Depending on the style and instructor, yoga can be very stress-reducing and rejuvenating.

Many books and magazines give different guidelines to the amount and type of exercise that is best. Usually no single exercise will fully meet your body's needs, although some like swimming come close. The American College of Sports Medicine recommends that healthy people work out, at a minimum, from three to five times a week, exercising at least 15 minutes to an hour without resting, at from 60 percent to 90 percent of the maximum age-adjusted heart rate. People with higher heart disease risk would start at a lower percentage of maximum heart rate and as their condition reversed, gradually increase their heart rate. It isn't usually necessary to go beyond 70 percent of your maximum heart rate to reverse heart disease.

Warming up and stretching are important parts of any workout in order to prepare the muscles for the extra demand and help prevent injuries. To get the most benefit from a workout, a cooling-down period is also recommended. Following a brisk walk, aerobic dancing, biking or any other high heart-rate activity, it is important to go a while at a slower pace, gradually reaching the resting point.

Many injuries occur from the lack of proper equipment. Walking and running shoes don't last as long as the tread designs on their bottom. The cushioning in the shoe absorbs most of the shock as the foot comes down to the surface, but the material has limited durability. A few months of use is a long time for running shoes, and in six months walking shoes usually no longer give the protection that is needed. In aerobics the floor surface can also be a source of injury. If the floor is hard, bring a piece of padded carpet or a mat to work on. When bicycling, wear a helmet with a label

showing ANSI and Snell approval. A proper helmet is a
cheap insurance policy. Why work for a healthy heart if you
don't protect against head injuries? Any good bike shop will
help you adjust the height of the saddle and position of the
handlebars to give the best workout. Proper adjustments are
important to avoid strains and injuries.

If you are between 30 and 69, the following guide will
help you evaluate your aerobic fitness level. Measure an
exact mile course on level ground and see how long it takes
you to cover it, walking as fast as you can. Heart risk individuals note: if you feel discomfort or pain, slow down and
try again later.

If you find yourself in the Poor or Fair category, your cardiovascular activity—related heart disease risk factor is at a
critical level. At a minimum, try to attain the High Average
level.

Table 21.3. Fitness Level for One Mile Walk
(Ages 30-69)

Men min:sec	Fitness Level	Women min:sec
less than 10:12	Excellent	less than 11:40
10:13 - 11:42	Good	11:41 - 13:08
11:43 - 13:13	High Average	13:09 - 14:36
13:14 - 14:44	Low Average	14:37 - 16:04
14:45 - 16:23	Fair	16:05 - 17:31
16:25 and more	Poor	17:32 and more

Source: Dr. James Rippe, University of Massachusetts

Persons who exercise strenuously for periods longer than
an hour every day and who sweat heavily can create special body demands. In a prolonged workout many vitamins
and minerals are lost in perspiration. These are replaced by
eating vitamin- and mineral-rich foods. Competing athletes

and persons who work out long and hard, especially in hot and humid conditions, may benefit from additional intake of vitamins B_2, C, E, iron, calcium and zinc, but large doses are not needed. Supplements are not usually needed by persons following the recommendations given in this book.

■ 22

Stress

Anxiety, pressure and worry have been recorded as human concerns since the first writings of history, but only since the 1940s have their relationship to disease been popularly discussed. Since then, stress has been accused of causing almost every known disease or health problem. It is not clearly established whether stress is a direct cause of coronary artery disease and heart attacks or if it is a complication that adds to the risk when other factors are present. It *is* known that psychological stress can cause arteries to constrict and spasm and that effectively dealing with stress has a beneficial effect on both physical and emotional health.

There are many ways to handle stress. It's difficult to avoid many of the sources of stress that we are exposed to. We can't always change situations that are highly stressful at work, at home and even at play, as they are often beyond our control. *Healing Heart* support groups address the issue by learning how to better handle the stress we encounter. This places more emphasis on assuming control of our own lives. It puts the responsibility for dealing with stress on ourselves, the one force in this world we each have the power to change.

To deal with stress, we must first determine what its source is. There are many different kinds of stress, and any combination of them may affect us. On its simplest level, stress is any situation that makes demands on us that are greater than our capability to deal with at the time. This can affect us physically, when our efforts fail to accomplish what we attempt. It can also be psychological, when pressures can disturb our emotional balance. For some it may cause discomfort; for others it may lead to misery and helplessness; and for a few, the loss of their ability to function at all.

How we interpret a situation or problem usually determines the stress we experience. The same situation that one person considers pleasant can be threatening to another. Going to the top of a high open structure makes me uncomfortable, and as I get closer to the edge, I feel more anxious and can't wait to get back down to ground level. If I look down, I get even more uncomfortable, so I try to focus on anything other than the height. To another person, height may not be the slightest unnerving. It may even be enjoyable. We *can* learn how to look at stress-causing factors in different ways, training ourselves to be less affected by them. We can learn how to change the way we see ourselves as we relate to stressful conditions, reducing and even eliminating their influence.

One of the most common sources of stress is change. Most of us can remember the stress we went through during the physical and emotional changes in our teens. We saw our bodies change; demands were made on us emotionally and through added responsibility, obligations and more. Like it or not, change is part of life. Nothing is as stable or as permanent as we might prefer. A new boss, a new relationship, a new baby, a different assignment, a crippled car, a sudden new pain are changes that can threaten our delicate balance and can make us anxious. Even small changes can bring discomfort; the change of an actor in a TV program, a change in the taste of a food or soft drink, or a new pair of shoes. How we recognize and deal with these factors will determine how much stress they cause us. *Find out what is causing your stress and understand how you are reacting to it.*

In doing this kind of self-evaluation I found that I had been using *denial* to avoid recognizing causes of my stress. When I had to dash across a street or move large amounts of dirt in my garden, I had a cold tightening pressure in my chest. It hurt, but I didn't want to deal with the possibility of what it could be. So I quickly "forgot" it. When my physician asked me if I had any chest pains, I answered no. I told myself that I hadn't, that what I felt was a temporary muscle cramp or strain. It was my way of dealing (very poorly) with that stress. I was avoiding the problem. Denying reality could have cost me my life!

Avoidance can have many forms. When we shut off our feelings, hiding them from others and ourselves, we can pretend they don't exist. We focus on other things, occupy ourselves with things to keep us busy, or do things to get people to react to other aspects of our behavior (from positive ones like making ourselves useful and needed, to negative ones like being argumentative and hostile). Avoidance can be a positive way of dealing with some things, but it needs to be recognized and then examined to find out if our avoidance is productive in dealing with the stress. Some people use drugs, including alcohol and tobacco, or even abuse food, to cope with their distress or to try to hide from it. These mechanisms might be useful if they made the problem go away, but since they don't deal with the source of the stress, they may even make it worse. Dr. Jon Kabat-Zinn, professor of medicine at the Massachusetts Medical Center and founder of its stress-reduction clinic, says it well. "The healthy alternative to being caught up in this self-destructive pattern is to stop *reacting* to stress and start *responding* to it."

Back in the dawn of our civilization, stress factors were simple: confronting a large animal, a battle with another tribe, a fight for a warm cave. To react to threat, our body produces substances to keep us alert and keep our heart-beat and blood pressure elevated. When faced with a threat, our ancestors had the choice of either defending themselves or trying to get away from the threat as quickly as possible. This is called the *fight-or-flight* reaction. It was appropriate for situations that brought about stress at that time, but in the complex world we live in today, fight-or-flight may be inappropriate or even harmful. This reaction still happens automatically, and unless we train ourselves to find other ways to deal with threats, we often continue to react in an unproductive way.

Learning to respond appropriately to stress, rather than reacting, requires the ability to focus: to *center* one's consciousness. Like some forms of meditation, it is a skill that is built with practice, and becomes easier and more automatic with time. Replacing the immediate fight-or-flight reaction with an appropriate response requires being aware of your reactions as well as understanding their source. Being upset, losing your cool or wanting to take some kind of action is part of the reaction. It needs to be replaced with a calmer, more peaceful activity before it can be controlled. Centering on some regular, rhythmic activity is often a way to recover. Many people concentrate on their breathing, listening to the sound of each breath and concentrating on the lungs filling and emptying.

Imaging is another technique for preventing automatic reactions from taking control. As an unpleasant situation begins to fill you with discomfort, try picturing a particularly pleasant experience. I remember the feeling I had the first time I climbed to the top of a mountain and looked down at the clouds, waterfalls and shaded valleys below. It was a special moment, not just because I made it to the top, but because I was seeing it for the first time and for the joy it gave me. In everyone's life there are many experiences that when remembered and focused upon, will bring a feeling of peace or satisfaction. When you feel a negative reaction to stress coming on, choose a pleasant, soothing image and let yourself "go" to that place again.

The different images we tend to create for ourselves are a real barrier to understanding who we really are. Some people call these *roles,* since they are often not who we really are, but who we think we must be. The roles we play differ according to the demands made on us. As a parent, we may be the authority; as an employee, we may feel we are without power, that we cannot avoid being pushed around.

A good way to get a better handle on the various roles you take in a typical day is to write down all the "titles" you have. Son/daughter, sister/brother, parent, spouse, bread-winner, caretaker, patient, companion, worker, boss, tax-payer, repair person, messenger, chauffeur, listener, stabilizer, spender, buddy, fun-maker and more. After you have a list of your roles, write down what is required to assume each role. Is the authority part of being a parent something you have special skills in, or are you assuming a "posture," a pose to convince others (and maybe yourself) that you are capable in that role?

Often we assume roles to keep us from having to deal with our lack of confidence or ability in another role. People who let their jobs keep them away from home to the point where their spouses complain may be uncertain about their

role at home. For these people, the job role may be familiar, comfortable and rewarding, but that may not be the case
in other roles. Sometimes, when a role is unclear or uncomfortable, a person avoids it. The example of the husband
who comes home from work, watches TV, works on his car
or goes out for recreation with his friends, and never seems
to "be there" when he's at home, might be a case of not
accepting or feeling comfortable in the husband/parent role.
If a particular role gives a person power, the temptation to
stay in that place as much as possible may become like an
addiction. Power is much like a drug—the more one has,
the more one seems to need. Focusing more on how to
empower ourselves and less on the need to exert power
over others can often lower stress levels considerably.

Another interesting way to assess the roles we assume is
to ask others to let us know what roles they see us in.
Rather than have them tell you and risk an argument, you
might ask them to write these down. Ask them to describe
the way you perform these roles after they list them, with
all the positive and negative behaviors they find for you in
each role. Be sure you really want to hear this; sometimes
the information you get may add to your stress. Seeing the
difference between the way others see us and the way we
see ourselves can help us put our behavior in perspective.
Once you have a clearer idea of your roles, you can begin
to use that information to see how you deal with stress in
each role: whether you are reacting or responding. You can
use this information to learn better ways of reducing stress.

Interpersonal stress comes from the way we deal with others. Even though there is stress potential whenever we relate
with other people, research findings show that we live longer
and have less heart disease when we live with others than
when we are alone. Yet some people avoid relationships,
keeping as much to themselves as possible, perhaps because
some of their past interactions were unsuccessful. We all have

our strengths and weaknesses in interpersonal skills, and it is important to know that we can learn to improve them, leading to greater success and lower interpersonal stress.

There's a popular T-shirt that bears this caption: "Insanity is inherited—you get it from your children." This may give parents a smile, but most people believe much of our behavior is genetically determined. We pick up behavior patterns from our family and friends early in our lives, but they are more often learned than inherited. We do what we've seen others do, even though we may not realize what we have seen. Sometimes we continue these patterns even when we know they don't work. Ironically, when the way we deal with a machine isn't productive, we usually change our approach. Most of us are a lot less flexible when it comes to dealing with people, and as a result, we give ourselves unneeded stress.

When we see people who are commonly impolite, hostile or aggressive, we're usually seeing people who aren't secure about their own feelings and have a poor understanding of what is expected of them. They may feel a need to control the situation, even though they know they will get a negative reaction from others. As a form of interpersonal communication, it isn't functional or beneficial, but it may give them the feeling that they are in control. If we react, we play into their hands. If we respond without getting caught up in their behavior, we keep our own stress under control, and they find that their actions won't work with us.

Effective interpersonal communication also requires a willingness to listen to the other person. Not just to hear the words, but to consider the feelings, meanings and needs of others. In disputes when labor confronts management, both sides have a set picture of the other side, and they know what they want to give and take. At first, extreme positions are often adopted, but as the sides negotiate, they get closer to a compromise. The negotiators themselves are rarely as rigid as the people they represent. They might ask with sincere interest about the other negotiator's family and share news of their own. That doesn't mean they weaken their position or give anything away. Experienced negotiators know that differences between them will eventually be settled, so they seldom allow personal feelings to interfere. They can settle major issues without creating an additional burden of personal stress. We all can learn to deal with difficult issues with a minimum of stress. We have to learn how to *respond* appropriately rather than *react* emotionally.

"I Hate You!"

A powerful technique, *active listening,* comes from Dr. Thomas Gordon's "Effectiveness Training" courses. It simply means to summarize what you've heard the other person say and tell that person what you think you heard. In my private practice I remember a family with a young son who, when he was denied anything he wanted (in this case an expensive radio) would yell, "I hate you. I want a new family. I don't like anybody in this house. Nobody loves me. I want a new radio." I doubt if he had any idea what he was saying, except that he wanted the radio. He'd keep it up until they'd either give up—and give him what he wanted— or react in some way they would be sorry about later and then, perhaps out of guilt, give him the radio. After the parents understood how to *respond* to his attempts to get them to *react,* they learned to respond with statements like, "I understand you're upset that you can't have the radio." The boy's puzzled response to that was, "I sure want that radio." Seeing that there would be no reaction, he went off peacefully to play with something else. The parents did not have to give in to his demands, did not scold him for wanting something expensive, and avoided conflict that might have led to bad feelings on both sides. The emotional climate in their home became much more comfortable for everyone.

Often our words, especially when emotions are high, are inflammatory reactions. They can escalate into damaging exchanges and are likely to bring fiery words that will be later regretted. Instead of dealing with the issues that caused the emotions, the emotional reactions themselves burn and scar, often taking the focus from the issue that set it off. An extinguisher is needed at that time, sounding something like, "I never looked at it that way before. Let me think about it," or "You've got a really good point there" and "Let's work together on this. We can probably settle it." Controlling the flames is not always possible, but fires that are not fed with fuel soon burn themselves out. You can usually avoid escalating the situation by keeping quiet or possibly going (calmly and courteously) to another room.

I remember having a person become even angrier at me when I said, "I'm sorry, I hadn't looked at it from your point of view before." When I asked her later why she got even madder when I apologized, she said that she had her arguments all ready and was frustrated when she didn't get to use them. We have to be ready to back down, take what is offered, and go on from there. A rigid position is often a reflection of a rigid person. When the stress of the wind pushes it, the tree that doesn't bend, breaks. We can learn to be like bamboo, to bend when pushed, and survive.

Job stress is much like any other kind of stress, except we may deal with it in different ways. When things get so difficult at work that we can't handle it, we may develop "injuries" and "illnesses" that keep us away. When we face stress at work, we may feel we have to accept it to protect our job and continue to earn a living. We may complain to our friends, family and co-workers, but the stress remains unchanged. At times, some of this stress may be intentionally caused by bosses who believe that they can get more from their workers when employees are uncertain and uncomfortable. To effectively deal with job stress, the first step is to identify the source of the pressure. Next, a list of potential ways to relieve the problem (and the possible consequences of doing so) can be made. Consulting with others who care about what happens to you is helpful in choosing any plan of action (which can include doing nothing).

Americans have another type of stress that is less often found in other parts of the world: our preoccupation with *time*. To many, there isn't enough time in the day to get everything done. Others can't find enough to do to fill their day. Almost everybody wears a watch. Many people wear one 24 hours a day, even in the shower or while sleeping. As strange as it seems, a good way to deal with not having enough time is to set aside a portion of your day for doing absolutely nothing. That doesn't mean sitting down and thinking about all the things you have to do or what you'd like to do, but doing and thinking *absolutely nothing*. If that sounds impossible, you might benefit from a class in meditation because that is a process meditation teaches.

The Power of Stress

A patient was sent to me who developed a paralysis of his right arm. He had been a bricklayer for 35 years, but years of drinking had caught up with him and he could no longer lay a straight line of bricks. He wasn't getting much work and he knew he wasn't doing a good job. One day he awoke and found he couldn't raise his right arm above his waist. When X rays and other tests found no reason for his paralysis, he was sent to me for diagnosis and recommendations. After exploring his feelings, emotions and concerns, I convinced his union to hire him as a job site inspector, a job he did well. Within a month he had gradually regained the full use of his arm. He had not been faking. His stress had been so great that his body reacted, causing his paralysis. Headaches, back pain and other disabling conditions can have stress as their source.

We often add stress to our lives by letting the events of the world affect us. Stories in the newspaper, on TV or the radio can make us angry, anxious and confused. We often forget that we have control over the on-off switch—we don't have to let these stories bother us. For a day with less stress, try a suggestion of Dr. Andrew Weil in his book *Spontaneous Healing*. Take a "newsfast."

Avoid all news sources, radio, TV, newspapers and news-magazines for the whole day. You can still read the comics and other fun features, but let go of the news. (The world will be pretty much the same tomorrow, even without you knowing what happened.) If your one-day newsfast made you feel better or lowered your stress level, try it once every week. You can later increase it to twice a week—or as many days a week as you like.

To become aware of the types of stress you encounter and how you are dealing with them, you can keep a list of all the stressful events of the day. A pocket-size notebook is a good place to enter them. Instead of waiting until later and possibly forgetting many important situations, you should jot down each episode as it occurs for at least a week. As you later look over your list, you'll recognize patterns of behavior that you never noticed before. It can help you to focus on the situations that need to be dealt with differently, and the patterns will often indicate the way to change. If you find a number of different things you'd like to modify, choose only one and work on that until you feel you've made progress; then go on to a second area. Don't try to deal with more than one at a time.

If you don't have enough time to learn how to deal with stress, and to center your awareness to bring you a sense of calm, and to revitalize your mind and body, will you have enough time later to be taken by ambulance to a hospital, to spend days there and weeks at home recovering from that heart attack or stroke? A few minutes invested now may pay dividends for a lifetime.

When you start to get caught up in the rat race, this thought may help put life in perspective:

The past is gone,
The future is yet to be.
Today is a gift—
That's why we call it
The Present.

23

Meditation

One of the most commonly misunderstood techniques for reducing stress and gaining inner peace is meditation. For many, the word meditation evokes an image of a "long-bearded guru" or a flower child of the 1960s, suggesting that "normal" people don't do these things. If "normal" means being overloaded with stress and not being aware of all the things that really matter to us, then the term "normal" may describe people who have not experienced meditation.

Most people go through a large part of their day without being fully aware of what they are involved in. We may eat while watching TV or reading, absently shoveling food into our mouths without being aware of the texture, taste and fragrance of what we're eating. We might answer another person's question while reading or watching TV, but if we were asked to repeat the question later, we'd have a hard time recalling it. We are seldom fully aware of what is going on around us, and we may be even less aware of our own being.

Our brain is constantly engaged in complex mental activity, but we are seldom aware of it. Meditation allows us to focus on our personal universe, to be conscious of the moment. By concentrating on something—perhaps a flower, a candle, a sound or word, or our breath—the number of randomly occurring thoughts decreases. Distractions, and our preoccupation with them, progressively become less frequent. Eventually, random thoughts just fall through, no longer interfering. The meditator may get caught up in a persistent thought pattern, but once aware of this, attention is gently brought back to the object of concentration. In time, meditation can also be objectless.

A deep meditation will permit the mind to become clear, uncluttered, focused and fresh. Not all meditations may be very deep, but with regular practice, the effects of meditation accumulate and become easier and deeper. The calm of meditation, along with stability and a clarity of focus, begins to carry over more and more into other daily activities.

For some people, meditation may be a spiritual practice, but it is not a religion. Meditation can be part of the of practice of religion, as in Hinduism and Buddhism. There are many biblical references to meditation. Churches usually have a meditative atmosphere. Meditation lets us connect with something within us that is peaceful, calm and refreshing, and that has some special meaning. Anyone can benefit from it, regardless of personal or religious beliefs.

Meditation is not the same as relaxation. Meditation *is* relaxing and much more. Relaxing can assume many forms, such as taking a hot bath or reclining in a soft chair and watching TV. The active process of meditation allows the body to relax and can offset the effects of mental and physical stress far more than passive relaxation. Thinking consumes energy. Constant thought activity, particularly random thinking, can result in headaches or feeling tired. The singular focus of meditation has the opposite effect.

In a small way, meditation is like self-hypnosis. The difference is that in hypnosis there is no attempt to maintain an awareness of the here-and-now, or to stay conscious of the process.

The first step is usually focusing on something to take your attention away from the random thought activity constantly going on in your head. This can involve concentrating on your breath, a solid object, a candle flame, a flower, a mantra (a phrase or word continuously repeated), or guided visualization. Some people use pictures such as a mandala, a highly colored symmetric painting. Others repeat mantras, with sounds that have a flowing, meditative quality and may be spoken out loud or repeated inwardly. Additionally, guided visualization is considered by some to be a form of meditation. A guided visualization, where another person directs your focus, can help to bring you into a meditative state. Visualization may also be used once a meditative state has been reached to achieve specific objectives. Audiotapes of guided visualizations are listed in the Recommended Resources section.

Some meditation techniques may work better for you than others. There is no "right" technique for everybody. The important thing is to find the way that works best for you.

Almost all of us have meditated at one time or another, even though we may not have been aware of it. If you have relaxed your thoughts while looking at a beautiful sunset, allowing your thoughts to quiet down, you have been close to meditation. After reading for a while, when you put the book down to take a break, sitting quietly and peacefully for a few minutes without thinking about anything, you are approaching a form of meditation.

Experienced meditators agree that early morning is one of the best times to meditate. In the early morning, worries, obligations and distractions usually haven't started to accumulate, so it is easier to establish a meditative atmosphere. Having an early morning meditation allows you to carry some of the energy and peace of the meditation into the rest of the day's activities.

Many people meditate either before dinner or later in the evening, too. Others also meditate at noon. A short meditation at these times provides a chance to get rid of some of the accumulated stress of the workday and become refreshed. Whenever your schedule will allow you to meditate is a good time, but having a special time of the day set aside for meditation can be especially helpful.

When first learning meditation, it is usually not possible to meditate for more than 10 minutes or so. After regular practice, it becomes easier to meditate for longer periods of time. Some people meditate twice daily for 20 to 30 minutes each time, but the right duration and frequency is for each individual to decide. More time is not necessarily better; most people consider a single daily 15-minute meditation sufficient.

To get the most from meditation try to do it:

♥ every day, preferably at the same time;
♥ not after eating a large meal;
♥ in a quiet place used for nothing else but meditation;
♥ with the spine straight and vertical (against a wall or in a chair for support).

Some people may find meditation relatively easy but find it harder to actually make themselves sit down and start their meditation. Soft, meditative music can help establish a conducive atmosphere.

The most common physiological effects of meditation are reduced blood pressure, lower pulse rate, decreased metabolic rate and other beneficial physical and chemical changes in the body.

Although it is possible to learn how to meditate from a book, most people who practice meditation agree that a teacher can be an important part of learning a meditation technique and making sure it is practiced correctly. The beginner will usually have several questions that only a teacher will be able to answer. Also, learning with other people in a meditation class gives the experience of group meditation, resulting in exceptionally powerful meditations for some people.

There are many individuals and groups teaching meditation. Different techniques are available, some more spiritual in nature and others mainly concerned with stress reduction and gaining peace of mind. To find the best one for you, sample a variety of approaches and teachers until you find one that works and is comfortable. Many instructors allow prospective students to visit a class without charge or for a small fee.

Audio and video tapes are available that teach and perfect all levels of meditation. A list of some recommended tapes is in the Recommended Resources section. Two books helpful to persons wanting to use meditation to lower heart disease risk are Jon Kabat-Zinn's *Full Catastrophe Living* and *Dr. Dean Ornish's Program for Reversing Heart Disease.* Each devote over 100 pages to meditation skills that can be learned and practiced at home.

24

Yoga

One form of stress reducing exercise that also helps people get in better touch with their body is yoga. It may sound a bit strange at first, but if reducing stress is your goal, especially if you have not found much help in other ways, it might be worth your time to try yoga. There are many physical benefits to yoga besides the reduction of stress. The sense of balance we tend to lose as we get older is often restored, and a feeling of confidence and well-being often comes to many other areas of our lives.

The Sanskrit word *yög(uh)* has two roots, *to meditate* and *to join* (as in combining human nature with forces beyond the body). The goal is to find a higher level of understanding of ourselves and of the natural world around us. Yoga is not always easily accepted in the Western world, as it extends beyond the limits of medicine as it is commonly practiced. What is not understood, or doesn't fit our usual pattern of knowledge, is often rejected.

Drawings illustrating yoga from 6,000 years ago have been found, but the full force of its influence on life in India goes back to about 300 B.C. Yoga is not just the physical poses that most people associate with it; it involves relaxation, breathing, diet and conscious awareness, a form of meditation.

In the Western world many different groups have been interested in Eastern ways of finding physical and emotional realization. Some have adopted yoga and given it religious significance, but yoga is not a religion in itself. It has instead been part of the search for understanding and inner peace practiced in many beliefs, especially Hinduism and Buddhism in the East.

There are four major forms of yoga. Physical mastery (hatha) is most popularly associated with what most Westerners know as yoga. In addition, there is mind discipline (laya), focus of thought (dhayna), and the control of knowledge, activity, psychic nerve forces and self-knowledge, leading to deep inner satisfaction (raja).

Hatha yoga, as well as the other forms, can aid many physical problems. Instead of concentrating on only increasing muscle size and strength, yoga also looks at finding ways of relaxing and stretching muscles to become more supple and responsive. It is a form of meditation with movement, with conscious awareness always focused.

Yoga allows people who have health problems to regain a sense of the power of their body. When a person has an illness, injury or physical problem, there's a tendency to become afraid or unwilling to fully utilize the body. What starts as a behavior to protect the body from injury can become the entire way a person lives, shaping that person's self-image. "I can't do that because I'm out of shape" is more a self-limitation, a lack of confidence (in mind and body), than an actual inability to perform a task or movement. We've all heard of persons lifting impossibly heavy objects to free a child or loved one. At the moment of a life-and-death emergency that person "forgets" about all the limitations that were self-imposed and without hesitation can do what was thought to be impossible. Yoga lets us get back in touch with our body, and that allows us to free our thoughts and emotions from the limits we have mistakenly imposed upon ourselves.

Yoga is a gentle form of exercise. It is not normally aerobic, and does not place a strain on the heart or other organs. A wide variety of yoga positions can be done in bed, sitting down, lying on the floor or standing. Many wheelchair patients are able to use yoga, and they find that it frees them from the disabled mentality that may have been holding back their recovery. Yoga becomes a rejuvenating process; the more it is practiced, the more energy is developed.

Yoga classes are available in most communities, some free and others for a small fee. Many adult education services, colleges and universities offer yoga. Classes are usually open to the general public as well as to students.

If these are not convenient for you, audio and video tapes provide carefully stepped introductions to the basic poses. To see if you might benefit from a video tape, a Jane Fonda Workout series low-impact yoga tape is available at many rental outlets. Some poses can place your back and body in alignment positions that you may not be used to, so it is best, at least in the beginning, to have an experienced yoga instructor guide you into the proper positions. It is possible to lose the benefits of the pose, and even to cause injury, if poses are done incorrectly. A list of selected training tapes and books about yoga is included in the "Recommended Resources" section.

READER/CUSTOMER CARE SURVEY

If you are enjoying this book, please help us serve you better and meet your changing needs by taking a few minutes to complete this survey. Please fold it & drop it in the mail. **As a thank you, we will send you a gift.**

Name: _____

Address: _____

_____

Tel. # _____

(1) Gender: 1) ____ Female 2) ____ Male

(2) Age: 1)____ 18-25 4)____ 46-55
2)____ 26-35 5)____ 56-65
3)____ 36-45 6)____ 65+

(3) Marital status:

1)____ Married 3)____ Single 5)____ Widowed
2)____ Divorced 4)____ Partner

(4) Is this book: 1)____ Purchased for self?
2)____ Purchased for others?
3)____ Received as gift?

(5) How did you find out about this book?

1)____ Catalog 2)____ Store Display
Newspaper
3)____ Best Seller List
4)____ Article/Book Review
5)____ Advertisement
Magazine
6)____ Feature Article
7)____ Book Review
8)____ Advertisement
9)____ Word of Mouth
A)____ T.V./Talk Show (Specify) _____
B)____ Radio/Talk Show (Specify) _____
C)____ Professional Referral _____
D)____ Other (Specify) _____

(6) What subject areas do you enjoy reading most? (Rank in order of enjoyment)

1)____ Women's Issues/ 5)____ New Age/
Relationships Altern. Healing
2)____ Business Self Help 6)____ Aging
3)____ Soul/Spirituality/ 7)____ Parenting
Inspiration 8)____ Diet/Nutrition/
4)____ Recovery Exercise/Health

(14) What do you look for when choosing a personal growth book?

(Rank in order of importance)
1)____ Subject 3)____ Author
2)____ Title 4)____ Price
Cover Design 5)____ In Store Location

(19) When do you buy books?

(Rank in order of importance)
1)____ Christmas
2)____ Valentine's Day
3)____ Birthday
4)____ Mother's Day
5)____ Other (Specify _____

(23) Where do you buy your books?

(Rank in order of frequency of purchases)
1)____ Bookstore 6)____ Gift Store
2)____ Price Club 7)____ Book Club
3)____ Department Store 8)____ Mail Order
4)____ Supermarket/ 9)____ T.V. Shopping
Drug Store A)____ Airport
5)____ Health Food Store

Which book are you currently reading? _____

Additional comments you would like to make to help us serve you better.

_____

_____

Thank You !!

NO POSTAGE
NECESSARY
IF MAILED
IN THE
UNITED STATES

BUSINESS REPLY MAIL
FIRST CLASS MAIL PERMIT NO 45 DEERFIELD BEACH, FL

POSTAGE WILL BE PAID BY ADDRESSEE

HEALTH COMMUNICATIONS
3201 SW 15TH STREET
DEERFIELD BEACH, FL 33442-9875

APPENDIX A

Understanding the Meaning of Laboratory Tests and Heart Disease Risk

Participants in *Healing Heart* support groups are requested to have some laboratory tests done as they begin the program and then repeat these tests at the end of the 10-week program. They can decide on the basis of changes in test results and the way they feel whether the lifestyle changes were worth the effort. Almost all have chosen to keep the changes, rather than return to their former lifestyle and problems. You are encouraged to do the same, getting your lipids, blood pressure, weight and body fat measured at the start and again at the end of 10 weeks. Seeing the numbers change for the better is proof that the program is working for you. But what do those numbers mean? The following is a limited, brief explanation to help give you basic understanding of the meaning and normal values of these tests. For more information, ask your physician for an interpretation of your test results.

The *cholesterol level* in your blood is a highly useful indicator in your health profile. It is measured in the U.S. in milligrams per deciliter (mg/dl).* The typical level of total serum cholesterol (the amount most commonly found in Americans) is somewhere between 130 and 350 mg/dl, with the average around 215. *To reduce plaque and heart attack risk, you should keep your cholesterol under 150.* Cholesterol levels provide information about many risks. If your cholesterol level is near the 215 average mark, your lifetime risk of heart disease and stroke is greater by 50 percent, of gallbladder disease 40 percent (90 percent of gallstones are made out of cholesterol), of breast cancer in women 10 percent, and of colon cancer 5 percent. Even small changes can have huge effects. Raising your cholesterol level from 200 to 260 increases the risk of dying from heart disease by 500 percent.

Cholesterol measures have a high margin for error. A reading of 200 can be anywhere from 185 to 215. It is best to use an average of three measures, rather than relying on a single one.

In addition to *total serum* (blood) cholesterol, there are three lipoproteins that give useful information. *High density lipoprotein* (HDL) is often called "good" cholesterol. The typical range in Americans is between 29 and 77. Any measure above 55 mg/dl is considered acceptable, but levels closer to 100 are related to a lower chance of coronary artery disease. A *heart risk ratio* is calculated by dividing total cholesterol by HDL. As total cholesterol is lowered, HDL will also often decline, sometimes causing the ratio to rise. This is not always a cause for serious concern, as the ratio has less significance as the total cholesterol level gets closer to 150. See the Risk Factor for an interpretation of the ratio.

---

*Cholesterol is measured outside the U.S. in millimoles per liter (mm/l). It can be converted to the U.S. measure by dividing by 0.0259. You can convert U.S. levels to the international standard by multiplying 0.0259 x mg/dl).

Low density lipoprotein (LDL) cholesterol, often called "bad" cholesterol, is useful in assessing heart disease risk, but many physicians feel it is not nearly as important as the total cholesterol and HDL counts. The typical level in the U.S. is between 75 and 185. It is considered beneficial to keep LDL levels under 130, as higher levels are associated with greater risk.

Some labs also calculate *very low density lipoproteins* (VLDL). The typical range is from zero to 40 mg/dl. The link between VLDL and heart disease risk is less well established.

Body fat percent is a way to determine the proportion of fat to other tissue. When fats are reduced and exercise increased, sometimes weight doesn't drop as expected. The fatty tissue may be replaced with newly formed muscle cells, which weigh more than fat. It is helpful to know the percent of fat in the body that is being reduced, even if weight sometimes doesn't change as much as expected. A general guide to body fat percentage is shown in the table below:

Table A.1. Body Fat Percentage

Men				AGE	Women			
Exclt	Good	Fair	Poor		Exclt	Good	Fair	Poor
10.8	14.9	19.0	23.3	**20-24**	18.9	22.1	25.0	29.6
12.8	16.5	20.3	24.3	**25-29**	18.9	22.0	25.4	29.8
14.5	18.0	21.5	25.2	**30-34**	19.7	22.7	26.4	30.5
16.1	19.3	22.6	26.1	**35-39**	21.0	24.0	27.7	31.5
17.5	20.5	23.6	26.9	**40-44**	22.6	25.6	29.3	32.8
18.6	21.5	24.5	27.6	**45-49**	24.3	27.3	30.9	34.1
19.8	22.7	25.6	28.7	**50-54**	26.6	29.7	33.1	36.2
20.2	23.2	26.2	29.3	**55-59**	27.4	30.7	34.0	37.3
20.3	23.5	26.7	29.8	**60+**	27.6	31.0	34.4	38.0

Source: National Dietary Research, Washington, D.C.

Triglycerides are the amounts of fats in your bloodstream. Since triglycerides usually go up after eating, a test for triglycerides should be taken only following 14 hours of fasting, eating no foods and drinking nothing but water. The typical triglyceride level is between 35 and 219 mg/dl, and levels below 100 are considered helpful in reducing heart disease risks. Triglyceride levels are somewhat different for men and women, and also change with age, rising to nearly double the value of age 6 by age 60. Then they slowly decline. Triglyceride levels commonly go up for three to six months when on a low-fat, vegetarian diet. They usually go below the starting level for much improvement after that. Fats in the blood rise to the top like the fats in soups or gravies do after they cool. If people who eat the typically high-fat standard American diet could see their blood sample after eight hours, with its layer of yellow-white fat floating above the red and sticking to the sides of the glass tube, it would be easier to motivate them to eat more sensibly.

Blood pressure is measured in two numbers. The higher number, called *systolic,* shows the highest amount of pressure on the walls of blood vessels during each beat of the heart. The lower number, *diastolic,* shows the amount of pressure on the arteries when the heart is resting between beats.

Various things can temporarily affect blood pressure, so it is usually best to take an average of many measurements rather than use only one. When some people go to a clinic, their anxiety can raise blood pressure much higher than normal, a condition called "white-coat hypertension." Recent use of coffee or tobacco can raise blood pressure. Many medications can raise or lower blood pressure.

Age, health problems and physical fitness are considerations when deciding if a person's blood pressure is normal. A general guide is given here, but you should check with your physician to decide if yours is safe or requires attention.

The following two tables show what are generally considered normal and high levels of blood pressure. Many different health conditions and medications may affect what is normal for each person.

Table A.2. Diastolic Pressure

Level Hg/mm	Significance	Usual Recommendation
85 & below	normal	check every 2 years
85-89	high-normal	check annually
90-104	mild hypertension	check 2 months later
105-114	moderate hypertension	medical intervention
115+	severe hypertension	therapy may be advised

When diastolic pressure is normal, a condition called isolated systolic hypertension may occur if systolic measures are abnormally high. This is more common in older persons.

Table A.3. Systolic Pressure
(When Diastolic Is under 90)

Level Hg/mm	Significance	Usual Recommendation
140 & below	normal	check every 2 years
140 - 159	borderline	check 2 months later
160 - 199	hypertension	consult your physician
200+	acute hypertension	therapy may be advised

APPENDIX B

Calories Burned
for Common Activities

—∿— In the following table, to find how many calories are burned during each activity, (1) multiply your exact weight by the number in the per pound column, then (2) multiply by the number of minutes in that activity. For example, a 162-pound person mowing a lawn burns .051 calories per pound, or 8.26 calories a minute. In a 45-minute session, this person would burn 372 calories. The same person, watching TV (sitting) for 45 minutes, burns less than 66 calories. Figures are shown for four weight levels, but you can easily calculate your exact rate. As you can see, body weight determines the number of calories burned; be cautious of any device or chart that does not use weight as a factor.

Table B.1. Calories Burned

Activity	per lb	Calories Burned per Minute			
		130 lb	150 lb	180 lb	210 lb
Sitting still	.009	1.17	1.35	1.62	1.83
Cooking	.022	2.86	3.30	3.96	4.62
Raking leaves, carpentry	.025	3.25	3.75	4.50	5.25
Grocery shopping, fishing	.028	3.64	4.20	5.04	5.88
Weeding	.033	4.29	4.95	5.95	6.93
Walking on a sidewalk	.036	4.68	5.40	6.48	7.56
Golf	.038	4.94	5.70	6.84	7.98
Weight training	.042	5.46	6.30	7.36	8.82
Bicycling 9.5 mph, aerobics	.045	5.85	6.75	8.10	9.45
Mowing the lawn	.051	6.63	7.65	9.18	10.71
Swimming, fast	.075	9.75	11.25	13.50	15.75
Running (9-minute mile)	.087	11.31	13.05	15.66	18.27
Running (6-minute mile)	.115	14.95	17.25	20.70	24.15

APPENDIX C

Living
with Omnivores

$-\wedge-$ When your spouse, partner or roommate doesn't
want to share your dietary restrictions, here
are some suggestions that have worked for many others.

Each person can prepare meals separately. While this
doesn't make for togetherness, it takes care of meals without any dietary sacrifice on the part of either person. The
time it takes to cook and prepare food is doubled, so unless
one of you is willing to cook and then wait, it usually
means eating separately. There's a potential positive,
though. If the person who doesn't want to eat very-low-fat
(VLF)/veggie foods isn't used to preparing meals, or doesn't
particularly like to cook, the tendency will be for that person to gradually start accepting (and often preferring) the
VLF/veggie meals as prepared. A word of advice: don't nag.
Don't even talk about food unless asked. Do your thing
with good grace and humor, without any hint of gloating,
superiority, guilt-making or resentment. Watch your body

language as well as verbal messages.

Alternatively, you can prepare two versions of each meal, one VLF/veggie and one containing the stuff the omnivore wants. It is surprising how many dishes can be prepared VLF/veggie first, reserving a portion for yourself, and then adding the *other stuff* to satisfy the other person. Love may be defined in many ways, but letting others do their own thing is one facet of making relationships work. Preparing carnivore foods may be a serious test of your limits; if this is too difficult, talk it out.

One VLF/veggie meal can be prepared and the omnivore can supplement it by adding other foods. A balanced VLF/veggie meal is available, but if the omnivore wants meat or higher-fat items, the option to add them is there.

A successful technique may involve a bit of deception. Using meat substitutes (see TVP and gluten/seitan in the Recipes introduction), you can prepare meals that appear to have meat or other expected ingredients but are truly meatless and low-fat. This approach is most successful when used occasionally, gradually becoming more frequent. After such a meal has been awarded a compliment, you can disclose that it was meatless. If no positive comment was made about the meal, or it wasn't well liked, it might be best to say nothing about the substitutes used. The usual reaction is one of surprise, disbelief and, finally, approval.

When a VLF/veggie dish gets compliments from your partner, serve it again after a short wait. If you can get some "favorite" dishes established, it will be easier for your partner to accept the other low-fat, meatless dishes.

An equitable basis of giving up things is to trade the elimination of vices. "I'll give up X if you give up Y." We all have some habits others see as negative (usually after the urgency of newly found love wanes). Caffeine or other health hazards are reasonable trades, as are habits that may be just annoying to your partner (knuckle crunching, tooth-picking, etc.)

Don't expect a person who is used to eating meat and who doesn't believe that a meal is complete without it to accept the transition in a short time. The change does happen, but it may take quite a while. A good way to make it happen is to set a positive example. If your attitude is bright and cheerful, your energy level higher, your affection undiminished and your health improved after not eating what your partner believes to be essential, gradually the realization that meat or fat is not necessary will settle in. Don't press, nag, or make sarcastic comments, and never criticize your partner's eating. When your mate isn't feeling well, is overtired, depressed or sluggish, don't fall into the temptation of saying "I told you so" or "If you'd just eaten . . ."

Having heard from many low-fat veggie/omnivore partnerships, it is clear that the desired change does take place in most cases, although sometimes more slowly than was hoped for.

When it comes to family, all reasonable wisdom may fail. If the other approaches don't convince them, and your conscience allows it, fibbing may be the most effective survival technique. If you can get your mate to support you, you can claim that you're allergic to the "enzymes in red meat" or a "protein factor in animal flesh" and may keel over or be messily sick within minutes after ingesting these. It may get you some strange looks and "See, I told you he/she wasn't the right one" attitudes, but there will be fewer arguments and much less chance of hidden meat or fats added with the belief that you'll never know the difference.

The most important thing is that you maintain your healthful eating style. If others around you choose not to follow the healthful patterns you have established, they will have to take responsibility for their own choices. Don't let others browbeat or ridicule you into changing what is best for you.

APPENDIX D

Dietary Fiber (Grams) in Common Foods

Table D.1. Dietary Fiber

Group	Food Item	Serving	Fiber (g)
Vegetables	kidney beans, cooked	half cup	6.9
and	pinto beans, cooked	half cup	5.9
Legumes	lentils, cooked	half cup	5.2
	green peas, cooked	half cup	4.3
	broccoli, cooked	half cup	2.4
	potato, raw, with skin	half cup	1.5
	tomato, raw	1 medium	1.0
Fruit	pear, with skin	1 large	5.8
	figs, dried	3 medium	4.6
	apricots, with skin	4 small	3.5
	apple, with skin	1 small	2.8
	banana	1 small	2.2
Grains	oat bran, dry	third cup	4.0
	oatmeal, dry	third cup	2.7

brown rice, cooked	half cup	2.4
white rice, cooked	half cup	0.8
whole wheat bread	one slice	1.5
white bread	one slice	0.6

Source: *Fiber Value from Plant Fiber in Foods, Second Edition.* Anderson, James W., M.D., Nutritive Research Foundation, Inc., P. O. Box 22124, Lexington, KY 40522.

APPENDIX E

Iron Content of
Some Plant Foods

Table E.1. Iron Content

	Food Ratio*	Portion	Iron (mg)
Swiss chard	11.3	1 cup	4.0
Blackstrap molasses	7.6	1 tblsp	6.4
Tofu, firm	7.1-9.9	½ cup	7-13
Beet greens	7.0	1 cup	2.7
Spinach	6.75	1 cup	2.0
Bok choy (Chinese cabbage)	5.6	1 cup	1.8
Turnip greens	4.0	1 cup	3.2
Tomato juice, canned	3.4	1 cup	1.4
Green beans	3.2	1 cup	1.1
Brussel sprouts	3.1	1 cup	1.2
Soybeans, boiled	3.0	1 cup	8.8
Broccoli	3.0	1 cup	1.1
Lentils	2.9	1 cup	6.6
Kale	2.8	1 cup	1.2

Quinoa, whole or ground	2.5	1 cup	5.3
Kidney beans	2.3	1 cup	5.2
Lima beans	2.1	1 cup	2.3
Pinto beans	1.9	1 cup	1.9
Peas	1.8	1 cup	2.5
Soy milk	1.8	1 cup	1.5
Prune juice	1.7	1 cup	3.0
Black beans	1.6	1 cup	3.6
Apricots	1.3	5 halves	2.0
Peas, blackeye	1.3	1 cup	4.3
Bulgur wheat, cooked	1.2	1 cup	1.8
Tempeh (soy product)	1.1	1 cup	3.8
Potato (medium size)	1.1	6 oz	2.8
Chickpeas/garbanzo beans	1.0	1 cup	4.7
Figs, dried	0.9	5 medium	2.1
Raisins	0.7	½ cup	1.6
Prunes	0.7	5 medium	1.0
Millet	0.5	1 cup	1.5
Watermelon	0.5	medium slice	1.6
Wheat gluten/seitan	0.1	½ cup	4.0

Source: *Composition of Foods,* USDA Handbook 8.
* The ratio is a measure of a nutrient per calorie. Many foods cannot be accurately measured as called for in recipes. Is a cup of spinach loosely or tightly packed? The ratio column lists milligrams per 100 calories of each food item, a constant value no matter what the portion size.

APPENDIX F

Common Plant Sources of Calcium

Table F.1. Calcium Content

Food	Ratio*	Serving	Calcium (mg)
Amaranth	857.1	1 cup	90
Turnip	684.0	1 cup	200
Collard greens	583.0	1 cup	355
Bok choy (Chinese cabbage)	511.0	1 cup	250
Mustard greens	490.5	1 cup	150
Seaweed, kombu (kelp)	391.0	½ cup	170
Seaweed, waka me, raw	332.8	½ cup	150
Blackstrap molasses	321.0	1 tablespoon	140
Kale	225.0	1 cup	200
Okra	197.3	1 cup	90
Broccoli	171.5	1 cup	180
Tofu, firm	141.6	½ cup	130
Squash, acorn	78.3	1 cup	90
Tortilla, corn	62.5	1 item	120

Baked beans, vegetarian	58.9	1 cup	130
Soybeans	58.7	1 cup	175
Great Northern beans	57.6	1 cup	140
Kidney beans	53.0	1 cup	115
Navy beans, boiled	49.4	1 cup	90
Figs	48.6	5 figs	135

* The ratio is a measure of a nutrient per calorie. Many foods cannot be accurately measured as called for in recipes. Is a cup of spinach loosely or tightly packed? The ratio column lists milligrams per 100 calories of each food item, a constant value no matter what the portion size.

Position of the American Dietetic Association: Vegetarian Diets

A considerable body of scientific data suggests positive relationships between vegetarian diets and risk reduction for several chronic degenerative diseases and conditions, including obesity, coronary artery disease, hypertension, diabetes mellitus, and some types of cancer.

Position Statement

It is the position of the American Dietetic Association that vegetarian diets are healthful and nutritionally adequate when appropriately planned.

Vegetarianism in Perspective

There is no single vegetarian eating pattern. The vegetarian diet is mainly plant foods: fruits, vegetables, legumes, grains, seeds, and nuts. Eggs, dairy products, or both may be included as well. The lactovegetarian diet is fruits, vegetables, grains, dairy foods, and their products, whereas the lacto-ovo-vegetarian diet also adds eggs. The vegan, or total vegetarian, diet completely excludes meat, fish, fowl, eggs, and dairy products. Even within specific classifications of the diet, considerable variation may exist in the extent to which animal products are avoided. Therefore, individual assessment is required in order to accurately evaluate the nutritional quality of a given diet. Studies of vegetarians indicate that they often have lower mortality rates from several chronic degenerative diseases than do nonvegetarians.[1,2] These effects may be attributable to diet as well as to other lifestyle characteristics such as maintaining desirable weight, regular physical activity, and abstinence from smoking, alcohol, and illicit drugs.

In addition to possible health advantages, other considerations that may lead to the adoption of a vegetarian diet include environmental or ecological concerns, world hunger issues, economic reasons, philosophical or ethical reasons, and religious beliefs.

Implications for Health Promotion

Mortality from coronary artery disease is lower in vegetarians than in nonvegetarians.[1,2] Total serum cholesterol and low-density lipoprotein cholesterol levels are usually lower, whereas high density lipoprotein cholesterol and triglyceride levels vary, depending on the type of vegetarian diet followed.[3,4] Low-fat, low-cholesterol vegetarian diets may decrease levels of apoproteins A, B, and E; alter platelet composition and platelet function; and decrease plasma viscosity. One study demonstrated reversal of even severe coronary artery disease without the use of lipid lowering drugs by using a combination of a vegetarian diet deriving less than 10 percent of its energy from fat, smoking cessation, stress management, and moderate exercise.[3] Vegetarians have lower rates of hypertension[5] and non-insulin-dependent diabetes mellitus than do nonvegetarians; lessening these risk factors may also decrease the risk of cardiovascular and coronary artery disease in the vegetarian population.

Seventh-Day Adventist vegetarians have lower rates of mortality from colon cancer than the general population.[6] This may be attributable to dietary differences that include increased fiber intake; decreased intake of total fat, saturated fat, cholesterol, and caffeine; increased intake of fruits and vegetables; and, in lactovegetarians, increased intakes of calcium. The dietary differences, especially in vegans, may produce physiologic changes that may inhibit the causal chain for colon cancer.[7] Reduced consumption of meat and animal protein has also been associated with decreased colon cancer in some, but not all, studies of omnivores. Lung cancer rates are lower in vegetarians, chiefly because they usually do not smoke, but possibly also because of diet.[8] Research suggests that vegetarians are also at decreased risk for breast cancer.[9]

Obesity, a major public health problem in the United States, exacerbates or complicates many diseases. Vegetarians, especially vegans, often have weights that are closer to desirable weights than do nonvegetarians.[10]

Vegetarians may be at lower risk for non-insulin-dependent diabetes because they are leaner than non-vegetarians. Also, vegetarians' high intake of complex carbohydrates, which are often relatively high in fiber content, improves carbohydrate metabolism and may lower basal blood glucose levels.[11]

Nutrition Considerations

Plant sources of protein alone can provide adequate amounts of the essential and nonessential amino acids, assuming that dietary protein sources from plants are reasonably varied and that caloric intake is sufficient to meet energy needs. Whole grains, legumes, vegetables, seeds, and nuts all contain essential and nonessential amino acids. Conscious combining of these foods within a given meal, as the complementary protein dictum suggests, is unnecessary. Additionally, soy protein has been shown to be nutritionally equivalent in protein value to proteins of animal origin and, thus, can serve as the sole source of protein intake if desired.[12]

Table G.1. Suggested Daily Servings

Food group	Suggested daily servings	Serving sizes
Breads, cereals, rice, and pasta	6 or more	1 slice bread, 2 buns, bagel, or English muffin 1/2 cup cooked cereal, rice, or pasta, 1 oz dry cereal
Vegetables	4 or more	1/2 cup cooked or 1 cup raw
Legumes	up to 3	1/2 cup cooked beans and other 4 oz tofu or tempeh
Meat substitutes		8 oz soy milk 2 Tbsp nuts or seeds*
Fruits	3 or more	1 piece fresh fruit 3/4 cup fruit juice 1/2 cup canned or cooked fruit
Dairy products	Optional—up to 3 servings daily	1 cup low-fat or skim milk 1 cup low-fat or nonfat yogurt 1 1/2 oz low-fat cheese

Eggs	Optional—limit to 3 to 4 yolks per week	1 egg or 2 egg whites
Fats, sweets, and alcohol beverages	Go easy on these foods and candies	Oil, margarine, and mayonnaise Cakes, cookies, pies, pastries Beer, wine, and distilled spirits

*These tend to be high in fat, so use sparingly if you are following a low-fat diet.

Daily food guide for vegetarians. Source: *Eating Well—The Vegetarian Way*. Chicago, Ill: American Dietetic Association; 1992.

Although most vegetarian diets meet or exceed the Recommended Dietary Allowances[15] for protein, they often provide less protein than nonvegetarian diets. This lower protein intake may be associated with better calcium retention in vegetarians and improved kidney function in individuals with prior kidney damage. Further, lower protein intakes may result in a lower fat intake with its inherent advantages, because foods high in protein are frequently high in fat also.

Plant carbohydrates are usually accompanied by liberal amounts of dietary fiber. This is in contrast to animal products, which are devoid of fiber. Fiber has been shown to be important in the prevention and treatment of certain conditions and diseases.

Vegetarian diets that are low in animal products are typically lower than nonvegetarian diets in total fat, saturated fat, and cholesterol, factors associated with reduced risk of coronary artery disease and some forms of cancer.

Adequate iron nutriture depends on both the amount of dietary iron consumed and the amount absorbed. Inhibitors and enhancers affect the absorption of nonheme iron, the form of iron found in plants. However, inhibitors and enhancers can offset each other when a variety of foods is consumed. Vegetarians are not at greater risk of iron deficiency than nonvegetarians, but Western vegetarians generally have better iron status than those in developing countries. Western vegetarians generally have an adequate intake of iron from plant products. They also consume greater amounts of ascorbic acid, an important enhancer of nonheme iron absorption. In contrast, vegetarians in developing countries rely on food staples that are low in iron; consume less ascorbic acid; and consume more tea, which contains tannin, an inhibitor of iron absorption.

The Recommended Dietary Allowance[13] for vitamin B_{12} is minute. Vitamin B_{12} is produced by microorganisms present in the guts or gastrointestinal tracts of animals and human beings, as well as in dirt on the surface of unwashed plants. Vitamin B_{12} is found in all animal products; hence, a pattern that includes animal products such as milk bacteria produce vitamin B_{12} in the human gut, but it appears to be produced beyond the ileum, the site of vitamin B_{12} absorption in the intestine.[14]

Lack of intrinsic factor in the stomach, rather than diet, however, is the most common cause of vitamin B_{12} deficiency. Atrophic gastritis, with the consequent bacterial overgrowth of the upper gut, may also contribute to vitamin B_{12} deficiency, especially in the elderly. Plants provide no vitamin B_{12}. In countries where sanitation is poor, vegans may derive vitamin B_{12} from foods that are contaminated with microbes, organisms that produce the vitamin, such as on the surfaces of unwashed fruits or vegetables. In Western countries, however, where sanitary practices are better, the risk of vitamin B_{12} deficiency may be far greater.

Vegans should include a reliable source of the vitamin in their diets. Spirulina, seaweed, tempeh, and other fermented foods are not reliable sources of vitamin B_{12}. As much as 80 percent to 94 percent of the so-called vitamin B_{12} in these foods, as measured by microbiological assay, may be inactive analogs. Cyanocobalamin, the form of vitamin B_{12} that is physiologically active for human beings, is available from vitamin fortified foods such as some commercial breakfast cereals, soy beverages, some brands of nutritional yeast, and other products.

Certain plant constituents appear to inhibit the absorption of dietary calcium, but within the context of the total diet, this effect does not appear to be significant. Calcium from low-oxalate vegetable greens, such as kale, has been shown to be absorbed as well or better than calcium from cow's milk.[15] Calcium deficiency in vegetarians is rare, and there is little evidence to show that calcium intakes below the Dietary Allowance[13] cause major health problems in the vegetarian population. The relatively high U.S. recommendations for calcium intake, compared with those for populations consuming a more basic diet, are designed to compensate for the calciuric effect of high intakes of animal protein, which are customary in the United States. Studies have shown that vegetarians, on the other hand, absorb and retain more calcium from foods than do nonvegetarians.[16,17]

Zinc is necessary for proper growth and development. Good plant sources include grains, nuts and legumes. Western vegetarians usually have satisfactory zinc status.[18]

Groups with Special Needs

Infants, children, and adolescents who consume well-planned vegetarian diets can generally meet all of their nutritional requirements for growth.[19,20] Those who follow vegan or veganlike diets should consume a reliable source of vitamin B_{12} and should have a reliable source of vitamin D. Calcium, iron, and zinc intakes may also deserve special attention, although intakes are usually adequate when reasonable variety and adequate energy are consumed.

If exposure to sunlight is limited, the need for vitamin D should be assessed. Because vegan diets tend to be high in bulk, care should be taken to ensure that caloric intakes are sufficient to meet energy needs, particularly in infancy and during weaning. Both vegetarians and nonvegetarians whose infants are premature or solely breastfed beyond four to six months of age should provide supplements of vitamin D, if exposure to sunlight is inadequate, and iron from birth or at least by four to six months of age.[21]

Well-planned vegetarian diets can be adequate for pregnant and lactating women. Vegetarians and nonvegetarians alike are generally advised to take iron and folic acid supplements during pregnancy, although vegetarians frequently have greater intakes of those nutrients than do nonvegetarians. A regular source of vitamin B_{12} is recommended for vegans during pregnancy and lactation.[21,22] A vitamin D supplement should be taken by pregnant and lactating vegans if exposure to sunlight is inadequate. Consumption of a variety of foods and adequate energy will help ensure adequate intakes of calcium, iron, and zinc.

Meal Planning

In planning vegetarian diets of any type, one should choose a wide variety of foods and ensure that the caloric intake is adequate to meet energy needs.[23] Additionally, the following recommendations are in order.

- ♥ Keep the intake of low nutrient-dense foods, such as sweets and fatty foods, to a minimum.
- ♥ Choose whole or unrefined grain products, instead of refined products, whenever possible, or use fortified or enriched cereal products.
- ♥ Use a variety of fruits and vegetables, including a good food source of vitamin C.
- ♥ If milk or dairy products are consumed, use low-fat or nonfat varieties.

♥ Limit egg intake to 3 to 4 yolks per week.

♥ Vegans should have a reliable source of vitamin B_{12}, such as some fortified commercial breakfast cereals, fortified soy beverages, or a cyanocobalamin supplement. A vitamin supplement may be indicated if exposure to sunlight is limited.

♥ Vegetarian and nonvegetarian infants who are solely breastfed beyond 4 to 6 months of age should receive supplements of iron and vitamin D if exposure to sunlight is limited.

The Dietary Guidelines for Americans[24] recommend a reduction in fat intake and an increased consumption of fruits, vegetables, and whole grains. Well-planned vegetarian diets can effectively meet these guidelines and can be a health-supporting dietary alternative.

References

1. Burr ML, Butland BK. Heart disease in British vegetarians. Am J Clin Nutr. 1988;48:830-832.

2. Fraser GE. Determinants of ischemic heart disease in Seventh-Day Adventists: a review. Am J Clin Nutr. 1988;48:833-836.

3. Ornish D, Brown S, Scherwitz L, Billings J, Armstrong W, Ports T, McLanahan S, Kirkeeide R, Brand R, Gould KL. Can lifestyle changes reverse coronary heart disease? Lancet. 1990;336:129-133.

4. Kestin M, Rouse I, Correll R, Nestel P. Cardiovascular disease risk factors in free-living men: comparison of two prudent diets, one based on lactoovovegetarianism and the other allowing lean meat. Am J Clin Nutr. 1989;50:280-287.

5. Beilin LJ, Rouse IL, Armstrong BK, Margetts BM, Vandongen R. Vegetarian diet and blood pressure levels: incidental or causal association? Am J Clin Nutr. 1988;48:806-810.

6. Phillips R, Snowdon D. Association of meat and coffee use with cancers of the large bowel, breast, and prostate among Seventh-Day Adventists: preliminary results. Cancer Res. 1983;45 (suppl):2403-2408.

7. Turjiman N, Goodman GT, Jaeger B, Nair PP. Diet, nutrition intake and metabolism in populations at high and low risk for colon cancer: metabolism of bile acids. Am J Clin Nutr. 1984;4:937.

8. Colditz G, Stampfer M, Willet W. Diet and lung cancer: a review of the epidemiological evidence in humans. Arch Intern Med. 1987; 147:157.

9. Chen J, Campbell TC, Li J, Peto R. In: Diet, Life-style and Mortality in China. A Study of the Characteristics of 65 Counties. Oxford University Press, Cornell University Press, and the China People's Medical Publishing House; 1990.

10. Bergan JC, Brown PT. Nutritional status of "new" vegetarians. J Am Diet Assoc. 1980;76:151-155.

11. Nieman DC, Underwood BC, Sherman KM, Arabatzis K, Barbosa JC, Johnson M, Shultz TD. Dietary status of Seventh-Day Adventist vegetarian and non-vegetarian elderly women. J Am Diet Assoc. 1989;89:1763-1769.

12. Young VR. Soy protein in relation to human protein and amino acid nutrition. J Am Diet Assoc. 1991:91:828-835.

13. Food and Nutrition Board. Recommended Dietary Allowances. 10th ed. Washington, DC: National Academy Press; 1989.

14. Herbert V. Vitamin B_{12}: plant sources, requirements, assay. In: Mutch PB, Johnston PK, eds. First International Congress on Vegetarian Nutrition. Am J Clin Nutr. 1988;48:452.

15. Heaney R, Weaver C. Calcium absorption from kale. Am J Clin Nutr. 1990;51:656.

16. Zemel M. Calcium utilization: effect of varying level and source of dietary protein. Am J Clin Nutr. 1988;48:880.

17. Marsh A, Sanchez T, Michelsen O, Chaffee F, Fagal S. Vegetarian lifestyle and bone mineral density. Am J Clin Nutr. 1988;48:837-841.

18. Hambige K, Casey C, Krebs N. Zinc. In: Mertz W, ed. Trace Elements in Human and Animal Nutrition. Vol 2. 5th ed. Orlando, Fla: Academic Press; 1986.

19. Sabate J, Lindsted K, Harris R, Sanchez A. Attained height of lacto-ovo vegetarian children and adolescents. Eur J Clin Nutr. 1991;45:51-58.

20. O'Connell J, Dibley M, Sierra J, Wallace B, Marks J, Yip R. Growth of vegetarian children: the Farm study. Pediatrics. 1989;84:475-480.

21. Food and Nutrition Board, Institute of Medicine. Nutrition During Lactation. Washington, DC: National Academy Press; 1991.

22. Food and Nutrition Board, Institute of Medicine. Nutrition During Pregnancy. Washington, DC: National Academy Press; 1991.

23. Eating Well—The Vegetarian Way. Chicago, Ill: American Dietetic Association; 1992.

24. Nutrition and Your Health: Dietary Guidelines for Americans. 3rd ed. Washington, DC: US Dept of Agriculture and US Dept of Health and Human Services; 1990.

♥ ADA Position adopted by the House of Delegates on October 18, 1987, and reaffirmed on September 12, 1992. The update will be in effect until October 1997.

♥ Recognition is given to the following for their contributions:

Authors:
Suzanne Havala, MS, RD; Johanna Dwyer, DSc, RD

Reviewers:

Phyllis Acosta, RD; Patricia Johnston, DrPH, RD; Mary Clifford, RD; Vegetarian Nutrition dietetic practice group: Winston Craig, PhD, RD, and Virginia Messina, MPH, RD; Pediatric Nutrition dietetic practice group.

This position paper was published in the *Journal of the American Dietetic Association,* November 1993, Volume 93, Number 11.

APPENDIX H

A Healing Heart
Progress Table

—⌐⌐— If you want to improve your health, lower your risk of heart disease and heart attack, and lower your chances of many other health problems, you can accept a 10-week challenge to see how effective these recommended lifestyle changes are. You will begin to feel and see the difference in only a week or two. Important changes will be happening *inside* your body, too.

For this 10-week challenge, you will need to know what you started out with and where you are at the end. Get a lipids profile (cholesterol lab test) just before you begin, and again during the 10th week. Don't be too concerned with weight loss. Body-fat percentage is often a better measure than weight, since muscle—which weighs more—may replace fat. Many health food stores offer body-fat evaluations at no cost. Take your resting pulse first thing in the morning, *before* you get out of bed.

Copy this table and put it on your refrigerator door. It will help remind you of your goals (and may help you control any temptation to "cheat").

Table H.1. Body Measurements

Measure	Start / /	Week 3 / /	Week 7 / /	Finish / /
Weight				
Resting pulse				
Blood pressure				
Body fat %				
Total cholesterol				
HDL				
LDL				
VLDL				
Triglycerides				

APPENDIX I

Commonly Prescribed Medications

—ᴧ— Oral medications to treat cardiovascular conditions have become specialized and sophisticated since 1950, when they first became widely available. A simple description of the different types of medication and what they do is presented. For each category, commonly prescribed medications are listed by their generic name. Following the equal sign, many of the manufacturers' TRADE NAMES are given.

It is important to realize that your personal physician chooses your medication not only on the basis of your heart risk factor, but on all the other information about your total physical condition, including your gender, age and ethnic group. If you want to know why your doctor has chosen a particular set of medications for you, you should ask. Some physicians may resent being "second guessed" by a patient, but others will appreciate your interest.

You have a right and need to know what chemicals you

are told to put in your body, what their potential short-term side effects and long-term consequences are, and why they have been prescribed. This information is far more important than the possibility of temporarily annoying your doctor.

Beta blockers are believed to reduce blood pressure by reducing the output of blood from the heart or by blocking responses from beta nerve receptors, which send the heart messages to speed up and pump more vigorously. They also reduce heart muscle oxygen demand, lowering the chance of angina during exercise or physical activity. Black Americans do not seem to benefit as much as other ethnic groups from beta blockers. Patients who suffer asthma or have circulatory problems in their legs and hands are not usually given beta blockers. Some commonly prescribed beta blockers are: *acebutolol* = SECTRAL; *atenolol* = TENORMIN; *metoprolol* = LOPRESSOR; *nadolol* = COR-GARD; *pindolol* = VISKEN; *propranolol* = INDERAL.

Alpha blockers, short for alpha-adrenergic blocking agents, help dilate vessels and lower blood pressure by blocking alpha receptors, which promote constriction of arterioles. Working on the autonomic nervous system, they also inhibit norepinephrine, a hormone that raises blood pressure when we react to stress. Alpha blockers can reduce the heart's load in some situations. Commonly prescribed alpha blockers are: *doxazosin* = CARDURA; *prazosin* = MINIPRESS; *terazosin* = HYTRIN.

When the risk of heart attack is elevated, *calcium channel blockers* are often prescribed. These synthetic drugs block the flow of calcium, allowing muscles to contract, affecting the size of the blood vessels. They may also help prevent spasms of the coronary arteries, lessening the risk of heart attack. Commonly prescribed calcium channel blockers are: *diltiazem* = CARDIZEM/DILACOR; *nicardipine* = CARDENE; *nimodipine* = NIMOTOP; *verapamil* = CALAN/ ISOPTIN/VERELAN.

When other medications prove ineffective, sometimes a combination of alpha and beta blockers is used. A commonly prescribed *combination blocker* is: *labetalol* = NORMODYNE/TRANDATE. Some side effects such as nausea, indigestion and dizziness are reported, but these usually decrease after a while.

The 1970s saw a new class of drugs that prevent production of angiotensin II, a hormone that constricts blood vessels. Called *ACE* (angiotensin-converting enzyme) *inhibitors*, they control other hormones related to heart disease and those that relieve edema. This can improve blood flow to some organs and reduce the body's demand for blood during heart failure. They have been helpful in reducing blood pressure and help prolong life while managing symptoms in congestive heart failure. These drugs sometimes cause a coughing reaction. A note of caution: these medications may react with TAGAMET (*cimetidine*), which is available without prescription. Some commonly prescribed ACE inhibitors are: *captopril* = CAPOTEN; *enalapril* = VASOTEC; *lisinopril* = PRINIVIL/ZESTRIL.

Anticoagulants help prevent clots (and prevent the enlargement of those already formed) in the blood. These are also used for persons during and after heart surgery. A commonly prescribed anticoagulant is: *warfarin* = COUMADIN/PANWARFIN.

Platelets are cells that stick together and form clots, and *antiplatelets,* such as *dipyridamole* = PERSANTINE, are used to help reduce this tendency in cases where it becomes necessary. These drugs are often called blood thinners, but that name does not correctly describe their function. *Aspirin* is the most common of the antiplatelets.

Drugs that reduce fluid retention are called *diuretics.* These lower blood pressure by causing the kidneys to excrete more salt and water, which reduces blood volume. While these drugs are often effective in reducing hypertension they may cause a loss of potassium, which should be checked occasionally. There is also evidence that in some people, cholesterol or glucose levels may rise with the use of diuretics. Some commonly prescribed diuretics are: *chlorthalidone* = HYGROTON; *hydrochlorothiazide* = ESIDRIX/HYDRODI-URIL/ORETIC; *metolazone* = DIULO/ MYKROX/ZAROXO-LYN. A more powerful group, called loop diuretics, works on another part of the kidneys. A commonly prescribed loop diuretic is *furosemide* = LASIX.

Nitrates are one of the most commonly used medications when the threat of heart attack is present. Many patients are advised to carry a small pill (or a spray) to place under the tongue when angina starts. This drug eases the efforts of the left ventricle, dilates vessels and lowers blood pressure. It also reduces spasm of the coronary arteries. Nitrates are extremely fast acting, and can be the difference between life and death when a heart attack is starting. While they relieve angina, they often cause strong headaches, although these usually taper off in a short while. Commonly prescribed nitrates are: *nitroglycerin* = MINITRAN/NITROGARD/BITRO-BID/DEPONIT NTG; *isosorbide dinitrate* = ISORDIL /ISO-BID/SORBITRATE/DILITRATE-SR.

Often two or more of these drugs are prescribed for maximum effectiveness. Some of these have been combined into a single dose. The choice of a *combination medication* is a decision your physician makes based on your particular condition. Since there are multiple effects, directions should be followed exactly and they should not be taken at different doses without consulting your doctor. Their main advantage is the convenience of only having to take one pill, and they may be less expensive than the total of the individual costs. Commonly prescribed combinations are: *amiloride/hydrochlorothiazide* = MODURETIC; *clonidine/ hydrochlorothiazide* = COMBIPRES; *hydrochlorothiazide/reserpine* = HYDROPRES; *labetalol/hydrochlorothiazide* =

NORMOZIDE/TRANDATE HCT; *methyldopa/hydrochloro-thiazide* = ALDORIL; *enalapril/hydrochlorothiazide* = VASERETIC; *propranolol/hydrochlorothiazide* = INDERIDE; *reserpine/hydralizine/hydrohlorothiazide* = SER-AP-ES; *spironolactone/hydrochlorothiazide* = ALDACTAZIDE.

In addition to drugs that deal directly with heart and vessel functions, some medications lower the risk of heart attack by lowering blood cholesterol levels. Dietary changes are the most effective way to lower cholesterol for most people and these changes seldom have side effects, unlike medication. *Cholesterol-lowering drugs* should only be used after a sincere attempt has been made to reduce dietary cholesterol and fat intake for at least three months. These drugs should never be used in place of a modified diet, but only as a supplement. Cholesterol-lowering drugs have many side effects and can interfere with the actions of other medications. Full understanding of the effects and careful consideration of alternatives are advised before starting on these. Some commonly prescribed cholesterol-lowering agents are: *lovastatin* = MEVACOR; *probucol* = LORELCO; *cholestryamine* = QUESTRAN; *colestipol* = COLESTID; *gemfibrozil* = LOPID; *niacin, nicotinic acid* = NA-BID/ NIACELS/NACOR/NIAPLUS/NICO-LAR/NICOBID/SLO-NIACIN.

PART TWO

A Healthy Heart Cookbook: 66 Very Low-Fat Vegetarian Dishes

Starting Out on the New Lifestyle

—∿— Making radical lifestyle changes, especially in what you eat, means learning some new ways to do old things. Some of the foods and spices in these recipes may be new to you, others may be used in different ways. Because some items in these recipes are used primarily by persons concerned with their health, the place you are most likely to find them is in a health food store.

A whole new world of fascinating foods, bulk items and supplements will amaze you on your first visit to a health food store (sometimes called a natural food store). There are a few things you should plan on buying on your first visit, but don't try to buy everything on your initial shopping trip. A list of basic items follows.

Many items you'll find in packages are also available in bulk. Bulk items are almost always sold by weight, usually by the pound. Since the recipes call for measurements in spoonfuls and cups, you might want to keep that in mind when deciding how much to buy. I sometimes take a measuring cup along to see how many cups make up a pound of each item and then write that on the container. Bulk foods are measured into plastic bags, but to keep them from spoiling or attracting insects, it's best to repack all bulk foods in tightly sealed glass jars or durable plastic containers.

Finding a colony of industrious insects in your food, just as you go to add it to a recipe you've already half-prepared, can be disastrous. To keep grains and many other bulk items from attracting visitors that may want to feast on your foods or raise their family in it, you can freeze the product for about three days. This usually stops all insect growth. Some find that adding a bay leaf to each container discourages insects without affecting the flavor, but that method may not work all the time.

Organic vegetables and grains are grown without chemical pesticides, herbicides or fertilizers, and are usually grown in earth that has been free of these elements for a number of years. Organic farmers may use natural pesticides, but the levels used are carefully monitored. The California Organic Food Act of 1990 sets strict standards that many products, including many not grown in California, claim to meet. Organic vegetables are usually more expensive than those grown with chemical treatment, and often organically grown produce is better selected and more attractive, but there is not always a great deal of difference in taste. If you are concerned about the high levels of toxic and carcinogenic chemicals that may be in your foods, it may be worth it to pay the additional cost for organic. Whether you buy organic or not, it is advisable to soak and wash all fresh produce before cooking, and especially before eating any raw. By replacing animal proteins and fats with a variety of vegetables, whole grains, legumes and fruit, gains in health will more than offset possible hazards present in non-organically grown produce. The choice of organic versus regular is personal, and lowering the risk of heart disease is not directly dependent on that choice.

One of the hardest things for many to learn is that oils are not needed in cooking, baking or marinating. Onions, garlic and most vegetables can be sautéed in almost any liquid, such as water, vegetable stock, low-sodium soy sauce, wine or balsamic vinegar. The heat has to be lower and it takes a few minutes longer, but the results are just as delicious. Salad dressing without oil can be made following the same recipes, by just omitting the oil, and can be thickened with guar gum or agar powder, a clear and tasteless gelatin made from sea vegetables. A few spoonfuls dissolved in boiling water and then added to the vinegar and spices will give the thick texture of oil, but with none of the fat. For baking, unsweetened applesauce usually provides an excellent substitute for oil. Although most recipes come out fine without any oil or shortening, a commercial fat substitute called Wonderslim, made mostly of prunes, can also be used. A simple recipe to make your own oil substitute (that I call "Wunderthin") is included.

Eggs are called for in many recipes, but egg yolk is one of the highest cholesterol sources and egg white is high in animal protein. Egg Beaters and other "yellow" egg substitutes are made of nearly 100 percent egg whites with coloring and sodium added. There are egg substitutes available in health food stores that have no protein or animal products. EnerG, one of the brands made of potato and tapioca starches and non-fat leavening, can be whipped like egg whites or used in sauces, custards and baked goods.

Often people assume that low-fat vegetarian cooking is more expensive than the foods they had been eating. If you keep careful records of your food costs, you'll find that after a few early purchases to get you started, this healthy way of eating *will save you as much as 50 percent on your food bills.*

Table II.1. Symbols and Abbreviations

C	Cup = 8 fluid oz, 237 ml
T	Tablespoon = 3 t, 1/2 fluid oz, 15 ml
t	teaspoon = 5 ml
oz	ounce: dry = 28.35 grams, liquid = 31 ml
lb	pound = 16 oz, 454 grams
"	inch = 2.54 cm
CFF	Calories From Fat

Table II.2. Oven Temperature Conversion

Electric		Gas mark	Description
°Fahrenheit	°Centigrade		
225	110	1/4	very cool
250	130	1/2	
275	140	1	cool
300	150	2	
325	170	3	low/very moderate
350	180	4	moderate
375	190	5	
400	200	6	moderately hot
425	220	7	hot
450	240	8	very hot

The Basic Essentials

Most of things you'll need can be bought at any large food store, but some items are usually carried only by health food stores. You may find these items at your local market. If not, try a health food store. Bulk items, which you measure into bags and pay for by weight, are usually cheaper than packaged equivalents. On your first visit to a health food store, you may want to stock up on these:

Table II.3. Basic Foods

Name	Appearance	Information
Nutritional yeast*	yellow flakes or powder	cheese-like taste
Balsamic vinegar	dark liquid, in bottles	sweet, wine-like
Whole wheat flour	light brown flour	full fiber, nutrients
Buckwheat flour	medium brown flour	great for pancakes
Cornmeal, polenta	coarse ground, yellow	baked goods
Lentils	small, bean-like, colors	low-fat, quick
Whole wheat pita bread	tortilla taste	sandwiches, pizza
Blackstrap molasses	very dark and thick	minerals, vitamins
Soy milk or rice milk	carton, not refrigerated	buy *no-fat* or *lite*
Low-sodium soy sauce (shoyu, tamari)	dark brown liquid	adds salt flavor
Rolled or steel cut oats	look like oatmeal	quick as instant
Rice cakes	round, popcorn-like taste	low calorie, filling
Grape-Nuts	wheat granules	non-fat, cereal or baking
Corn Flakes	generic brands good	cereal and cooking
Active dry yeast	in envelopes or jar	homemade bread, pizza
Dried beans	black, pinto, kidney, Great Northern, garbanzo many more	stews, casseroles, Crock-Pot chili, salads

*Ask for and buy only a nutritional yeast that is fortified with vitamin B$_{12}$.

Spices will give you a variety of tastes and interesting new dishes. You may have many of these items already, but you'll need all of them to make the *Healthy Heart* recipes:

Table II.4. Spices

Dry mustard	Chili powder	Dried onions
Cumin	Black pepper	Thyme, ground
Oregano	Garlic powder	Turmeric
Basil	Celery seed, ground	Seasoned salt
Cinnamon	Sage, ground	Lite salt
Baking powder	Cocoa	Italian seasoning
Ginger, powdered	Paprika	Parsley, dried
Vanilla (or vanillin)	Mustard seed	Rosemary
Cornstarch/arrowroot	Dill, dried	Liquid smoke
Curry powder		

Buy green vegetables in small quantities and use them while they're fresh. Frozen vegetables have all the nutritional benefits of fresh produce, and since they are usually frozen within hours of being picked, may even be fresher than those that have taken days to reach your grocer. Canned vegetables have some of their vitamins and minerals cooked out of them and are usually high in sodium. Look at the ingredients and read the label for added oils and salt. Many vegetables can be grilled or barbecued, and can be marinated to add a variety of flavors.

Following the recipes is an introduction to some less well-known foods.

Cooking Methods

Many of these recipes can be cooked in a microwave oven. Cooking times suggested are for a 700 watt microwave, but the time needed varies greatly by manufacturer and age of the oven. Always use non-metallic cookware and cover, at least with a paper towel or plastic wrap, to avoid splattering and damage to the oven interior.

Conventional oven temperatures are given in degrees Fahrenheit.

For baking and stovetop cooking, high quality non-stick cookware is recommended. Some cheap non-stick pots and pans only retain their non-stick surface for a short time. Do *not* use non-stick sprays when baking with non-stick pans or dishes as this will coat them with a brown surface that is difficult to remove without damaging the non-stick surface, making them less efficient in the future. When using non-stick sprays, remember they are made mostly from fats. Spray a very small amount in the center and then spread with a paper towel.

Meat substitutes are available for most familiar cuts. Textured vegetable protein (TVP) comes in granules that taste like ground beef, and in chicken, pork or beef-like chunks excellent for stews and stir-fries. Gluten (seitan) and soy protein foods that resemble ham, pepperoni, corned beef, bologna, hot dogs and a number of fish and seafoods are available. Some of these are very high in fat while others are fat-free, so read labels carefully. Some are frozen or ready to eat, others come packaged to be mixed with water, stock or tofu. A few vegetarians are uncomfortable about eating meat analogs (foods that look or taste like animal products) while others use them as a transitional food as they move away from familiar meat dishes. These substitutes are a matter of personal choice, and are fine for reversing heart disease risks. They can solve the problem of what to serve to a meat-eating guest.

Introduction to the Recipes

All but one of the recipes in this cookbook follow the guidelines for not more than 10 percent calories from fat, and only a few have more than 15 percent of calories from protein. The oatburger patties are 12 percent calories from fat, but when a whole wheat bun and lettuce and tomato are combined with one, the sandwich is much less than 10 percent. The average of all recipes included is less than 7 percent calories from fat.

Each of these recipes was tested by, served to and approved by both omnivores and vegetarians. The serving sizes may be too large for some, far too small for others. Eating more than one portion only increases the number of calories; but there is no change in the proportion of fat, protein and carbohydrates. That's why you can eat all you want of the foods that meet the guidelines. In most cases, along with recommended aerobic exercise, many people can increase the amounts they eat and still lose weight. Diabetics and those who experience difficulty losing weight should limit their sugar intake. The nutritional program recommended here should not be considered a diet, but rather a change in the kinds of foods you eat.

These recipes come from a number of sources. Many of them were originated for the *Healing Heart* program; a few were suggested by support group participants themselves. A number of these were found on the Internet, a computer network. Repeated testing in the kitchen brought many modifications, sometimes changing things so much that the original recipes may no longer be recognized. These recipes are a way to get you started, examples of the variety and ease of preparing food that meets the guidelines. The names of books featuring low-fat vegetarian recipes can be found on page 290.

The nutritional analysis was done with the computer

program, *Nutritionist IV.* Within its database of nearly 10,000 food items, a breakdown of almost every important nutritional element is available. Only calories, grams of fat and the percentage of calories from fat, protein and carbohydrate are included here. Some nutritionists feel that fat can be averaged over the whole day, but a single meal high in fat can bring about significant changes in the body, and often will cause considerable discomfort to those who have been eating low fat for a while. It is recommended that the percentage of calories from fat be considered for each meal, and that you try to observe the 10 percent limit for every meal or snack.

To make it easier to follow while cooking, each recipe is on a separate page. *Healthy Heart Hints,* with tips for easier and simpler preparation, have been included where space permits. Some recipes will work for Crock-Pot-type slow cookers, but a large covered pot on very low heat will work just as well. The advantage of the Crock-Pot is that it can be prepared the night before or early in the morning, and without having to watch or stir it, the meal will be ready when you've returned at the end of a busy day.

I make large amounts of each of these recipes, many times the amount shown. After eating one portion, I put the remaining warm food in zip-seal sandwich bags, squeeze any air out, let them cool and lay them on a flat surface in the freezer. When frozen solid, I file them like books on the freezer shelves. They are ready for instant microwaving, a three-minute preparation dinner. I only cook full meals about twice a week, but every night I have a choice of dozens of entrées. Each bag is labeled with a permanent marking pen, showing the contents and date it was made. With such a wide variety of things available to eat, I'm not tempted to go out for fast food, even when I don't feel like cooking. There's always a hot meal about five minutes away, and no pots and pans to clean up. You'll be amazed at how easily dishes and cookware clean up when there's no fat or oil.

These recipes are well seasoned, but none are overly hot or spicy. After you've made a dish according to the recipe, try adding other spices or replacing some ingredients with others. Much of the fun of cooking is making things a little different each time, at least until you have them exactly the way you want them. A few people will feel these dishes are too bland. If they aren't tasty enough for you, add peppers or other stronger spices. For those who like things a bit less spicy, use less of the strong spices in the recipe. If a dish comes out too spicy for your taste, try mixing some beans or potatoes or non-fat soy milk into the dish. Often this will make strong flavors more mild. If it is still too spicy, freeze it, and the next time, make it without the strong spices and combine the frozen one with the new dish.

This special collection of recipes should get you started on a lifestyle that will improve health, provide more energy, help take off excess pounds and save as much as 50 percent of your food costs.

To expand your collection of low-fat vegetarian dishes, look for *Vegetarian Times* and other magazines featuring this lifestyle. Many communities have a vegetarian society that meets regularly and can provide valuable information, recipes, books, audiocassettes, videocassettes and inspiring speakers. Health food stores often can provide information about a group in your area.

BASICS

WUNDERTHIN

A fat and egg substitute for cooking,
baking and salad dressings

12 oz prunes	*3 T unbleached lecithin*
3 C water	*¼ t citric acid*

Cover prunes with water and bring to a boil. Cool. Blend with all other ingredients until smooth. Pour in a clean quart jar and refrigerate. Keeps about one month in the refrigerator; indefinitely in the freezer.

Wunderthin is Healing Heart's version of a commercial fat substitute made by Wonderslim. It is easy to make and has the same ingredients. The directions on the jar say that ¼ cup of the product replaces ½ cup of butter, oil or margarine. A one-for-one ratio may yield better results.

When cooking with Wunderthin, reduce the amount of sugar in the recipe, as there is natural sweetness in the prunes.

Makes about 3½ cups, or 14 ¼-cup servings. Very low sodium: 3.8 mg.

Per ¼ cup serving: Calories 76.6, Fat 0.74 (8.5% CFF), Carbohydrate 17.1 g, Protein 0.56 g.

HEALTHY HEART HINT:

♥ Unsweetened applesauce can be used to substitute for oil, butter or margarine in most baked goods. Use the same quantity applesauce as oil.

CHICK'N-STYLE SEASONING

When a recipe calls for vegetable or chicken broth,
use this seasoning mixed with water instead

1⅓ C nutritional yeast flakes   *1 t celery seed*
3 T onion powder   *3 T Italian seasoning (or 1½*
2½ t garlic powder   *T oregano + 1½ T basil)*
1 T salt   *2 T parsley, dried*

Put all ingredients except parsley in a blender and make a fine powder. Stir in parsley. Store in airtight container.

Making this yourself is much less expensive than buying vegetarian chicken broth. You'll find it tastes better and has much less salt.

You can use this seasoning to make a quick chicken-like stock out of water when you have no veggie stock on hand. Excellent for flavoring rice and as a soup base.

36 servings, 1 T each: Calories 21, Fat .049 g (2% CFF), Carbohydrate 2.85 g, Protein 2.16 g.

HEALTHY HEART HINT:

♥ To make a very simple, easy and tasty *gravy*, combine: 1 T Chick'n-Style Seasoning, 1½ cups water and 2 t miso. Just before serving, blend 1 to 2 T corn starch or potato starch in ¼ C water and add to gravy. Thicken over medium heat until you reach desired thickness.

GOLDEN CHEAZE SAUCE

Non-dairy and very low-fat, with a taste similar
to American or mild cheddar cheese,
it can be used as a cheese spread

1½ C Great Northern beans,
cooked (or one 15.5-oz can)
6 T nutritional yeast
¼ C pimiento pieces (or ¼
C chopped, cooked, sweet
red bell pepper)
Juice from one freshly
squeezed lemon

1 T low-salt *shoyu or tamari*
1 t onion powder (see below)
½ t any type of prepared
mustard
½ t salt

In a blender, mix all ingredients until very smooth.
Refrigerate and store in a sealed container.

You can spoon *Golden Cheaze* over baked potatoes (with
soy "bacon" bits), or use as a sauce over vegetables, as a
Welsh rabbit (add a little non-alcoholic beer and
Worcestershire sauce) or as a chili-con-queso when mixed
with salsa. Sprinkle over tacos and in enchiladas instead of
dairy cheeses. Heated with a little white wine and a pinch
of nutmeg, it makes a filling fondue, served with squares of
whole wheat French bread. Mix with a cup of corn kernels
and diced celery for a hearty corn and cheaze soup.

6 ½-cup servings, each: Calories 69, Fat 0.28 g (4% CFF),
Carbohydrate 12.25 g, Protein 5.01 g.

HEALTHY HEART HINT:

♥ A spin in a blender or coffee mill, and dried chopped
onions (flakes) become onion powder.

SNACKS

CRISPY BAKED ONION RINGS

Baked instead of fried,
these satisfy cravings without fat

2 large sweet onions
1 (7-oz) package Corn
  Flakes cereal, crushed
2 t sugar
1 t paprika
1 t seasoned salt (or a pinch
  of all-purpose seasonings,
  garlic powder and ¾ t salt)

1 C powdered egg substitute
  (in 2 C water)
Vegetable cooking spray
  (such as Pam)

Cut each onion into 4 thick slices; separate into rings, reserving small rings for other uses. Set aside.

Combine cereal, sugar, paprika and salt; divide in half, and set aside.

Beat egg substitute at high speed with an electric or hand mixer until soft peaks form. Divide onion, egg whip and cereal into two portions. Dip one portion of the onion rings in egg substitute foam, then dredge in crumb mixture. Place in a single layer on non-stick baking sheets *or* regular baking sheets very lightly coated with cooking spray.

Repeat procedure with other portion of onion rings, egg foam and crumb mixture. Bake at 375°F for 15 minutes or until crisp; serve warm. These do *not* save well; eat 'em now or forget 'em.

4 large servings, each: Calories 254, Fat 0.5 g (2% CFF), Carbohydrate 50.6 g, Protein 10.8 g.

PRETZELS

Choose large or small, salted or plain—
these can be a soft or crispy snack

2¼ t yeast (or one packet)	*4 C flour (see HINT below)*
1½ C very warm water	*1 T sugar*
(about 102°F)	*1 t salt*

Add yeast to warm water and stir until muddy. Add flour, sugar and salt. Mix and knead dough. Roll into a sheet and then cut in strips to make "ropes." Shape in traditional pretzel bows or roll to make sticks. Place on ungreased cookie sheet (1 second of a non-stick spray may be used). Bake at 425°F for 12 to 15 minutes, or until light brown.

For a special treat, just before baking, sprinkle some with garlic powder, chopped onion, any favorite herbs or spices, or—if sodium is not a problem—coarse salt.

Averages 18 pretzels, 12 to 15 large or 24+ smaller ones.

Each pretzel (of 18): Calories 94, Fat 0.5 g (4% CFF), Carbohydrate 20.2 g, Protein 3.8 g.

HEALTHY HEART HINT:

♥ When baking, use whole wheat, rye and oat flours and specialty grains instead of white flour for tasty and higher fiber treats. A mixture of ½ whole wheat and ½ white flour bakes much the same as white flour. White flour has most of its vitamins, minerals and fiber removed. Finer whole wheat pastry flour is less grainy.

POTATO PEARLS

These tasty appetizers can be prepared
in advance, frozen, then baked when needed

1 pound potatoes
½ C chives or green onions,
  finely chopped

Salt and pepper to taste
½ t paprika
½ C wheat germ

Preheat oven to 375°F. Cover potatoes with water and boil until soft. Peel and mash, adding onions, salt and pepper. Shape into 1-inch balls. Mix the paprika and wheat germ together in a dish and roll potato balls in mixture until coated. Coat baking sheet with 1 second of a non-stick spray and spread with a paper towel. Place potato balls on baking sheet, making sure they do not touch one another. Bake for about 20 minutes. Serve hot, a toothpick in each.

10 servings, each: Calories 54, Fat 0.64 g (10% CFF), Carbohydrate 10.02 g, Protein 2.46 g.

HEALTHY HEART HINT:

♥ Many foods that were formerly fried can be baked or broiled. Vegetables can be coated with a savory coating and heated till golden brown. For an easy "shake-bake" coating, mix ½ C corn flakes, finely crumbled; 1 t *lite* seasoned salt; ½ t each paprika, sage, onion powder; ¼ t each garlic powder, thyme, pepper. The foods to be coated can be moistened or dipped in a mixture of 4 T *EnerG* egg replacer and 8 T water that has been beaten to a foam. Bake at 375°F for 15 minutes or until browned and crispy. Serve and eat immediately.

TOMATO TANGO

Quick and easy as a side dish,
relish or summer salad

6 med. tomatoes, quartered
1 med. onion, sliced
1 med. green pepper,
  cut into strips
1 large cucumber, sliced
¾ C cider vinegar
¼ C water

1½ T sugar
1½ t celery salt
1½ t mustard seed
¼ t salt
½ t cayenne pepper (adjust
  to taste)
⅛ t black pepper

In a large bowl combine tomatoes, onion, green pepper and cucumber.

In small saucepan combine vinegar, water, sugar, celery salt, mustard seed, salt, cayenne pepper and black pepper. Bring to boil and then boil 1 minute. Pour hot vinegar mixture over tomato mixture.

Cover and refrigerate 8 hours to blend flavors.

4 servings, each: Calories 97, Fat 1.26 g (10% CFF), Carbohydrate 22.8 g, Protein 2.88 g.

HEALTHY HEART HINT:

♥ To get rid of the odor on your hands after slicing onion, garlic or other strong spices, wash your fingers with a small dab of toothpaste. A little scrubbed into your cutting board will help, too.

ASPARAGUS GUACAMOLE

Avocados are 90 percent fat—this
taste-alike is quick, easy and low fat

1 C cooked asparagus	*½ t cumin*
2 T diced chili peppers (or	*¼ t garlic powder*
less, according to taste)	*⅛ t white pepper*
2 t tomato paste	*(fine-ground black pepper*
2 t lemon juice	*can be substituted)*
1 T chopped onion	
3 T fat-free mayonnaise	
(without egg whites)	

Put all of the ingredients in a blender or food processor.
Blend to desired consistency.

Serve with fat-free baked tortilla chips, or make your own
corn chips by cutting corn tortillas into strips and baking in
325°F (warm) oven for about 20 minutes, or until crisp.

6 servings, each: Calories 16.2, Fat 0.21 g (10% CFF),
Carbohydrate 3.0 g, Protein 1.4 g.

HEALTHY HEART HINT:

♥ To make an easy thick, rich salsa, put 5 T chopped
dried onions in a 16 oz (pint) jar, add 1 t each of garlic powder, ground cumin, oregano, chopped green onion and
cilantro. Add hot sauce to taste. Fill jar with tomato juice;
shake; add more juice. Let sit overnight in the refrigerator.
Finely diced cucumber, celery and sweet bell peppers can
be added to taste. Use reduced-salt tomato juice for a
sweeter, fresher taste. Keeps three weeks if refrigerated.

ARTICHOKE AND TOMATO ALFREDO

Rich and creamy, but low in fat and calories.

*12 oz whole wheat fettuccini,
    macaroni or spaghetti*
1 medium onion
*4-5 fresh tomatoes, chopped
    into large chunks*
*2 cloves garlic, chopped fresh
    (or 1 T garlic powder)*
*½ C fresh basil, chopped
    (or 3 T dried basil)*

*1 can artichokes
    (not packed in oil)*
2 T whole wheat flour
*½ C (or more) non-fat
    Soy Moo or any low-fat
    soy or rice milk*

Prepare whole wheat fettuccini, macaroni or spaghetti noodles *al dente*.

Place onion, tomatoes, garlic and basil in a non-stick pan and sauté in a little of the liquid from the can of artichokes. Cut the artichokes into small pieces. Add the artichokes (and liquid) into the sauté with a little flour to thicken. Mix thoroughly, adding soy or rice milk and flour to desired thickness. Don't cook the artichokes for long—just enough to heat all ingredients and to blend sauce to desired thickness. Top the pasta with the artichoke sauce.

2 servings, each: Calories 210, Fat 1.5 g (6% CFF), Carbohydrate 46 g, Protein 10.7 g. (Pasta = 100 calories/cup.)

HEALTHY HEART HINT:

♥ Keep your spices in the dark. Light, as well as air, causes many spices to deteriorate. Spice racks may look good, but professional chefs keep their spices in light-proof, air tight containers.

CREAMY CORN BISQUE

A dairy-free, rich, thick and creamy soup,
or a main dish over brown rice, baked potato or pasta

1 pkg frozen corn or 2 ears
  fresh corn (salt-free
  canned corn can be used)
1 C onion
4 C water
low-salt *shoyu or tamari*
  to taste

¼ –½ C corn meal
2 stalks celery (if desired)
1 C favorite fresh or thawed
  frozen vegetables

Defrost the corn (if frozen) in water. Drain corn, saving water. Saute onion and corn in a little water (1 T low-salt shoyu or tamari adds flavor). Add ⅛ C corn meal, stirring so that all veggies are covered. Slowly add water, stirring to avoid lumps. Starting with ⅛ C, gradually add a little more corn meal, but wait before adding all—it thickens as it cooks. Bring to a boil, then simmer for about 30 minutes. Add celery and vegetables, and cook another 10 minutes. Salt or tamari can be added at any time during the process, but is best added (if at all) at the end. To serve over rice or pasta, add water to thin slightly.

6 servings, each: Calories 121, Fat 1.19 g (8% CFF), Carbohydrate 26.46 g, Protein 3.65 g.

HEALTHY HEART HINT:

♥ For a quick meal, microwave or bake a potato and cover it with your favorite thick soup, chili, salsa or sloppy joe. Baked potatoes can be frozen and thawed later.

BOSTON BAKED BEANS

A colonial favorite

*2 C (18 oz) dry Great
Northern beans (navy
beans can substitute)
1 T baking soda
1 large onion, chopped finely
2 T blackstrap molasses
⅓ C brown sugar*

*1½ t dry mustard
½ t liquid smoke or
1 t smoked yeast or
3 T artificial bacon bits
1 T soy sauce or tamari
1 bay leaf
1 clove garlic, minced*

Cover beans with water with 1 T baking soda added and soak overnight (or at least 5 hours). Rinse. Cook beans at low boil in 4 C water without salt for 1 hour. Drain, reserve liquid. In a heavy ceramic dish with lid, layer onion at the bottom, cover with beans.

In a separate container, mix all remaining ingredients and then pour over beans. Bake at 275°F for 3 hours, then stir well. Bake for at least 2 more hours or until beans are soft. If beans are too dry, add reserved liquid; if too wet, uncover for last half hour of baking. Remove bay leaf before serving.

4 servings, each: Calories 208, Fat 1.38 g (6% CFF), Carbohydrate 41.96 g, Protein 8.75 g.

HEALTHY HEART HINT:

♥ While some energy is saved by not preheating your oven (many ovens reach very high temperatures—far higher than the dial is set to—while preheating), most baked dishes will come out better when placed in an oven already at the right temperature.

QUICK FIXES

SLOPPY JOES

A treat for kids of all ages

1 large onion, chopped
1 to 2 C celery, chopped
1 t balsamic vinegar (other
vinegar may be used)
3 cloves garlic, crushed
(or 2 t dried minced
garlic or garlic powder)
1 green bell pepper, chopped
1 T chili powder (will not
make it too hot)
2 T cumin
2½ C tomato sauce (or a
6-oz can tomato paste + 1C
tomato juice + 1 C water)

1½ C dry TVP granules
1 T prepared yellow mustard
1 T ground dry mustard
1 T brown sugar
1 t blackstrap molasses
1½ C boiling water
Optional spicy version:
1 to 3 t hot sauce or
roasted chilies

In a medium pan, sauté onion and celery in balsamic vinegar and a little water on medium heat. Add more water if needed. Add garlic, peppers and spices and sauté for a few more minutes. Add everything else and simmer for 20 minutes. Serve over whole wheat buns, rice or pasta.

Adding a can of chili beans makes a very filling dish, changing it slightly to *Sloppy José*.

6 servings, each: Calories 152, Fat 1.85 g (10% CFF), Carbohydrate 19.86 g, Protein 17.44 g.

HEALTHY HEART HINT:

♥ Avoid high temperatures for dishes made without oil. Non-stick cookware will last longer and work better if high heat is avoided.

POTATO PANCAKES (LATKES)

Very low in fat, with no milk or eggs—
tastes like the traditional European recipe

2 T oat flour
(see HINT below)
¼ C water
¼ C onion, chopped
(or 4 T dried onion)

1½ C shredded potato
(can use frozen "Simply Potato")
Pinch of salt
Freshly ground black pepper (if desired)

Mix flour and water, add onions and potato. Add a bit more water if needed to form thick pancake batter.

In non-stick pan with a ½-second spray of Pam fry till golden brown with some darker spots. Add salt and pepper (optional) to taste.

Serve with unsweetened applesauce or preserves. Makes 4 large pancakes.

Each pancake: Calories 70.7, Fat 0.39 g (5% CFF), Carbohydrate 15.06 g, Protein 2.16.

HEALTHY HEART HINT:

♥ When a recipe calls for small amounts of oat flour, you can make it from rolled oats or oatmeal in a blender or electric coffee mill. Many other grains can be made into flour or breading mix this way.

LIMA LINGUINI DIABLO

Less than 10 minutes to the table

1 lb whole wheat linguini	*3 scallions, thinly sliced (or*
1½ C vegetable stock (or	*shallots, leeks, green onions)*
Chick'n-Style Seasoning	*3 T brown mustard (partially*
and water)	*ground, grainy-style is best)*
2 C frozen baby lima beans	*6 ripe tomatoes, seeded, sliced*

Prepare linguini *al dente* (just a little chewy) in large pot of boiling water, about 6 minutes. Drain. In another pot, while linguini is cooking, bring vegetable stock to a boil. Add lima beans, scallions and mustard. Slow boil for 7 minutes, add tomato slices and remove from heat. Pour over warm linguini and gently mix. For a creamier sauce, smooth half the beans in a blender and mix with the rest of the sauce.

6 servings, each: Calories 352.5, Fat 2.54 g (6% CFF), Carbohydrate 69.34 g, Protein 12.38 g.

HEALTHY HEART HINT:

♥ Vegetable stock is easy to make. Veggie bouillon cubes and powders for dissolving in water are available in health food stores and some supermarkets. Some products are high in salt, so read labels carefully. Making vegetable stock at home is simple: just put onions, garlic and your favorite vegetables, roots and greens in a pot, bring to a boil, then simmer for two hours. Strain. Try adding a bay leaf, some basil and other herbs. Stock keeps best frozen. Cubes are handy for sautéing; zip-seal bags for cup-size portions.

5-MINUTE BOK CHOY AND ORIENTAL MUSHROOMS

Quicker than calling for Chinese takeout

*1½ C vegetarian broth
(or Chick'n-Style
Seasoning and water)
1 green onion, sliced fine
1 large clove garlic, finely
chopped or pressed
2 T fresh ginger, finely
chopped or pressed
5 button or straw mushrooms,
cut if necessary*

*5 shiitake mushrooms, cut
into ½ inch pieces
(rehydrated or fresh,
no stems)
4 C bok choy, (Chinese
cabbage) chopped
(or 4 baby bok choy)
2 T cornstarch mixed
with ¼ C of cool water*

Pour broth into a skillet, add half the green onion, garlic and ginger. Sauté in broth—no oil—for a few minutes, and then add mushrooms.

In a covered dish, steam bok choy in a microwave for 2½ to 3 minutes, mixing and checking every minute. Bok choy can be prepared in a vegetable steamer if preferred.

Thicken the broth with cornstarch. Make it slightly thicker than looks right, as the moisture from the bok choy will thin it a bit as it cooks.

Toss in the bok choy and mix. Serve over rice, your favorite grain or a baked potato.

4 servings, each: Calories 60, Fat 0.64 g (9% CFF), Carbohydrate 9.5 g, Protein 5.2 g.

SEEDED ZUCCHINI STEAM-SAUTÉ

Flavors of three continents

*1 large carrot (about 6 oz),
cut in matchsticks or grated*
*3 large zucchini (about
1¼ lb), cut in matchsticks
or grated*
2 t chili powder*
*1 t mustard seed (black
mustard seed is preferred)*

1 t cumin seed
*1 small onion (about ¼ lb),
thinly sliced*
3 T vegetable stock or water
*Salt (or garlic salt) and
pepper to taste*

Toss together carrot, zucchini and chili powder in a medium bowl. Heat a medium-sized, non-stick skillet over high heat. Put mustard seed in the pan and cover immediately. Listen carefully when seeds begin to pop (holding the lid firmly on the pan). Swirl pan over the heat until popping dies down. This will take 2 to 3 minutes. Pour seeds into vegetable mix. Reduce heat to medium and put cumin seeds in the pan. Toast, swirling frequently, until the seeds become fragrant, about 2 minutes. Pour seeds onto vegetables and mix. Add onion to the pan, cover, and cook for 2 to 3 minutes until it begins to brown and stick to the pan. Add stock or water and stir onions to unstick and dissolve brown bits. Continue to cook and stir until liquid has evaporated and onion is limp. Add vegetable mixture and cook, stirring frequently, until tender-crisp—3 or 4 minutes for matchsticks, 2 minutes if grated. Season with salt and pepper, if desired, and serve.

6 servings, each: Calories 34, Fat 0.4 g (10% CFF), Carbohydrate 6.8 g, Protein 1.5 g.

---

*Chili powder does *not* make this dish highly spiced. If a very bland dish is preferred, use 1 t chili powder and taste test.

COLCANNON

A creamed kale, leeks and potato dish

4 medium or 3 large potatoes
1 onion
3½ C chopped kale
(one bunch)*
3 leeks

⅓ C non-fat Soy Moo or
any low-fat soy or rice milk
¼ C fresh parsley, chopped
Salt and freshly ground
pepper to taste

Cut up the potatoes and steam until soft (potatoes can be microwaved in a bowl with a little water for about 15 minutes). Meanwhile, chop the onion and sauté in a non-stick pan with a little water (no oil). Chop and wash the kale and leeks, and when the onion is soft, add the kale and leeks to the skillet. Cover and let the kale steam in the water that stays on the leaves after washing. When the potatoes are done, drain if necessary and mash (with or without the skin, as you prefer). Mix in the soy or rice milk, parsley, and salt and pepper to taste; combine with the kale and onions, and serve. Makes 3 large or 4 medium servings.

3 servings, each: Calories 262, Fat 1.2 g (4% CFF), Carbohydrate 57.6 g, Protein 8.3 g.

HEALTHY HEART HINT:

♥ Add salt at the end of cooking: you'll use much less and get the same taste. If a saltier taste is needed, sprinkle a little "lite" salt on the food when served.

---

*If kale is hard to find, most greens (mustard, turnip, collard) can be used. Cabbage is another traditional colcannon ingredient.

QUICK SOUTHWEST SKILLET DINNER

Colorful and tasty

1 onion, chopped
1 green bell pepper, chopped
2 cloves garlic, minced
2 T chili powder
½ t salt
½ t cumin
4 T water or wine
1 can tomatoes

1 can kidney beans
1 can corn or *1½ C*
    frozen corn
8 oz whole wheat elbow
    macaroni or other pasta,
    cooked
Hot sauce to taste

Sauté onion, green pepper, garlic, chili powder, salt and cumin in water or any red or white wine until vegetables are tender. Stir in tomatoes, breaking with spoon. Add kidney beans and corn; bring to a boil. Reduce heat and simmer 15 minutes, stirring occasionally. Toss with pasta.

Note: The chili powder does not make this dish hot, and should be added even by those who don't like spicy foods. There are two types of chili powder at most markets, the regular (mild) one and a hot Mexican-style chili powder. For a spicy dish, use the hot chili powder or add hot sauce.

4 servings, each: Calories 446, Fat 1.92 g (4% CFF), Carbohydrate 95.39 g, Protein 17.68 g.

HEALTHY HEART HINT:

♥ Fresh basil and other herbs, as well as fresh garlic and onions, make a tastier and much more fragrant dish. (If time and convenience prevent you from using fresh herbs, use dried ones.) If you enjoyed the dish, you'll like it even more with fresh ingredients.

SALADS
AND
SAUCES

CILANTRO CHUTNEY

1 bunch fresh cilantro
(also called Chinese
parsley or coriander)
1 t lemon juice

1 T raisins
¼ t salt (optional)
⅛ t artificial coconut
flavor (optional)

In a blender, mix all ingredients until smooth, adding water to desired consistency.

This sauce adds variety served over vegetables or rice dishes, and makes an interesting topping on baked potatoes.

4 servings, each: Calories 11, Fat .01 g (1% CFF), Carbohydrate 2.53 g, Protein .49 g.

HEALTHY HEART HINT:

♥ Chutneys are an Indian relish to accompany almost any dish, most commonly served with curry in the West. Mango chutney is a sweet-sour and often hot fruit preserve, but chutneys can be made of any fruit or vegetable, and sometimes with yogurt.

To make a fruit chutney, use 2 C of semi-ripe fruit (mango, nectarine, citrus), ⅓ C vinegar, 1 C sugar, 1 chili, ½ C raisins, ¼ C chopped onion, ⅛ t salt. Boil sugar and vinegar 5 minutes, add all other ingredients, slow cook 90 minutes. Seal in sterile jars or refrigerate.

AZTEC BEAN SALAD

Tasty but mild

1 onion, sliced
1 T chili powder (optional)
2 C cooked green beans
1 15-oz can black beans,
　drained and rinsed
1 15-oz can red kidney
　beans, drained and rinsed

1 15-oz can white beans,
　drained and rinsed
1½ C fresh or frozen corn,
　drained
2 T chopped cilantro or
　parsley
¼ C water

Cook onion in water until soft and separated into rings, about 4 or 5 minutes. Add the chili powder and mix well. Remove from heat. Combine all the ingredients in a large bowl and mix well. Cover and place in the refrigerator for at least 2 hours to bring out the flavors fully.

Serve with Aztec Accent (see recipe). Makes 4 complete meal servings or 6 to 8 salad or side dishes.

4 servings, each: Calories 447, Fat 2.27 g (5% CFF), Carbohydrate 84.34 g, Protein 27.61 g.

HEALTHY HEART HINT:

♥ Hot peppers contain capsaicin, which has been linked to lowering cholesterol and blood pressure and protecting against some forms of cancer. Capsaicin also releases endorphins in the body, relieving pain and bringing a feeling of peace and well-being. Even the hottest peppers become mellow and sweet when they are roasted. Roast large peppers on a cookie sheet under a broiler, watching carefully and removing them as they become dark brown. Put them in a paper bag to steam, then rinse and peel. Discard seeds, stems and ribs.

AZTEC ACCENT

A dip, a taco sauce, a salad dressing or
a seasoning for many other dishes

¼ C fresh cilantro, chopped
1 4-oz can green chilies,
  chopped
¼ C fresh lime juice
2 cloves garlic
1 T onion

2 t honey
½ t oregano
¼ t cumin
Black pepper, freshly
  ground, to taste
¼ C water

Place all of the ingredients in a food processor or blender.
Blend until smooth.

For a milder taste, peperoncini can be substituted for the
green chilies. Remove stems and seeds and save the pickling
juice for salad dressings, pasta sauces and other recipes.

To make a tangy and different salsa, add 2 medium fresh,
ripe chopped tomatoes to this recipe.

Refrigerate leftover sauce.

4 servings, each: Calories 48.3, Fat 0.13 g (2% CFF),
Carbohydrate 11.54 g, Protein 0.53 g.

HEALTHY HEART HINT:

♥ Many spices retain their flavor better when added near
the end of cooking. Unless the instructions say otherwise,
wait until the last 10 minutes before adding them. When
whole seeds are used as a spice, they should be "roasted"
by heating in a covered non-stick pan until they pop or
begin to release their fragrance.

SOUPS

SWEET AND
SOUR CABBAGE SOUP

A full meal in a bowl

⅓ C uncooked barley
1 large carrot, sliced
1 stalk celery, chopped
1 medium onion, chopped
2 bay leaves
4½ C water or vegetable
    stock
3 C red cabbage, coarsely
    chopped or shredded

1 14-oz can no-salt-added
    plum tomatoes and liquid
    or 10 fresh roasted tomatoes
    with skins
3 t red wine vinegar
2 T brown sugar or honey
2 t paprika
½ t dried thyme
Ground pepper and salt to taste

Place barley, carrot, celery, onion and bay leaves in large
pot and cover with 4½ cups water or vegetable stock. Bring
to boil and then add all remaining ingredients. Cover and
simmer over low heat for 30 to 35 minutes, or until veggies
and barley are tender. Allow soup to stand for an hour (to
blend flavors) and then heat before serving. Also good cold.
Makes 6 large bowls or 8 cups.

6 servings, each: Calories 95.5, Fat 0.57 g (5% CFF),
Carbohydrate 21.8 g, Protein 2.8 g.

HEALTHY HEART HINT:

♥ To bring out the full, rich flavor of tomatoes, instead
of boiling them, slice them in half and oven-bake them in
a deep-sided roasting pan at 375°F for about 25 minutes.
Let cool and pierce the skin with a knife, then gently peel
skins off.

LENTIL SOUP (SHORBAT ADTS)

This Middle-East dish is light but filling

2 C split red lentils
1 onion, chopped
1 small carrot, peeled and
  chopped
1 small zucchini (or ½
  large), chopped
2 cloves garlic, crushed

1 t coriander
2 t (or more) cumin
½ stalk celery, chopped
  (optional)
3 C vegetable broth or water
Salt and pepper to taste
Dash cinnamon (optional)

Boil all the ingredients over medium heat in 3 C veggie broth or water. Check every 10 minutes or so and add water as needed. It should take about 30 to 40 minutes before the lentils are soft and tender. Smooth in a blender and return to pot. Add 2 t (or more) cumin and 1 t of coriander, plus salt and pepper to taste. A dash of cinnamon adds a special taste. Cook about 5 to 10 minutes more. If too thick, add a little water. Serve with a lemon wedge and pita "croutons" (toast or dry out pita bread in the oven and break into pieces).

4 servings, each: Calories 143, Fat 0.2 g (2% CFF), Carbohydrate 27.6 g, Protein 8.1 g.

HEALTHY HEART HINT:

♥ This traditional Arabic dish is especially good with an Arabian Salad made of 2 chopped tomatoes, 1 peeled and chopped zucchini, ½ onion chopped very fine and several scallions.

Toss with 2 t cumin, a dash of coriander and a small sprinkle of cayenne, ½ T lemon juice, 1 t each vinegar and salt, and about a tablespoon of water. This salad is tastier if it sits awhile before serving. Serve at room temperature with pita bread and the soup, falafel or couscous.

ROMANY POTAGE

An Authentic Gypsy repast

1 can or 2 C cooked
   garbanzo beans
   (chick-peas)
1 can stewed tomatoes
1 large onion, chopped
2 large sweet potatoes or
   yams, cut in ½" cubes
1 large green pepper,
   chopped
½ C fresh or frozen corn
½ C fresh or frozen peas

1 C celery, chopped
3 cloves garlic, minced
   (or 2 t garlic powder)
2 t paprika
1 t turmeric
½ t cumin
½ t cinnamon
4 C water
½ t salt
Pinch of cayenne or other
   hot pepper

Blend or mash ½ the garbanzos. Add all ingredients in a large pot. Stir and cook until done, 45 minutes to an hour. Serve over rice or pasta, or as a thick soup with whole wheat sourdough bread.

4 servings, each: Calories 509, Fat 3.8 g (6% CFF), Carbohydrate 112.7 g, Protein 13.8 g.

HEALTHY HEART HINT:

♥ Canned beans and vegetables are very high in sodium. If you are cutting down on salt, try cooking your own beans. Soak overnight with a T of baking soda, rinse and slow cook until tender in 2 C water to 1 C beans. To quick-steam fresh or frozen vegetables, microwave in plastic wrap about 2 minutes per serving. Add ½ t or less water or soy sauce.

SAUERKRAUT SOUP SOVIET

Dr. Zhivago's favorite meal

*8 C vegetable broth
(or Chick'n-Style
Seasoning and water)
16-oz can or jar reduced-salt
sauerkraut
15-oz can low-salt tomato
sauce
2 turnips, peeled, cubed
(about 1 lb)*

*3 carrots, peeled, finely
chopped
1 onion, finely chopped
1 t caraway seed
Freshly ground pepper and
salt (optional) to taste*

Place all the ingredients in a large covered pot and bring to a boil. Reduce heat and cook for 1 hour. Serve hot with fresh bread. Can also be used as a sauce over brown rice or pasta if the amount of stock is reduced to 4 cups.

The original Russian recipe was high in fat and cholesterol. This adaptation retains the flavor, but is extremely low in fat and has no cholesterol. The caraway seeds are essential to bring out the traditional flavor in this dish.

8 servings, each: Calories 161, Fat: 0.23 g (2% CFF), Carbohydrate 28.32 g, Protein 4.81 g.

HEALTHY HEART HINT:

♥ It's wise to avoid most seeds and nuts, as they are very high in fat. Caraway seeds and the seeds of some green spice plants are exceptions. If you crave nuts, there is one that is very low-fat: the chestnut. Roasted chestnuts can be used to replace peanuts and cashews in many recipes, diced or finely ground. Before roasting (oven at 375°F for 15 to 20 minutes or microwave), cut an X on the flat side to prevent them from exploding. Buy chestnuts in season, roast, chop and freeze. They'll keep frozen until the next chestnut season.

MAIN MEALS

CHILI CHAPULTAPEC

People will swear there's meat in it

2 medium onions, chopped
1 green pepper, chopped
*   (vary amount to taste)*
1 T balsamic vinegar
1½ cans garbanzo beans
*   (chick-peas)*
2 cans dark red kidney
*   beans, drained (or black*
*   beans, if preferred)*
1 t chili powder

1 t paprika
1 t oregano
1 t cumin
1 t garlic powder
1 pinch turmeric
2 16-oz cans whole, peeled
*   tomatoes (or tomato pieces)*
1 C TVP granules (optional;
*   see below)*
Salt to taste

Sauté onions and green peppers in balsamic vinegar *(no oil)*. Drain and rinse beans, then, using a potato masher or large fork, mash all the garbanzos and half the dark red kidney beans. Add mashed beans to onions and peppers and cook for a few minutes. Add chili powder, the other spices, both cans of tomatoes (split tomatoes in your pot with the spatula) and the rest of the whole kidney beans. Simmer for at least 45 minutes, stirring occasionally. While simmering, test for the degree of "hotness" you prefer and add more chili powder to your taste.

This is a thick, rich chili because of the mashed garbanzos. If you'd like to add a traditional "ground meat" texture, add 1 C TVP (textured vegetable protein) granules and ¾ C water before simmering.

Serve with brown rice, or over split baked potatoes or pasta. Excellent in tacos or burritos.

4 servings, each: Calories 388, Fat 3.8 g (8% CFF), Carbohydrate 73.2 g, Protein 20.3 g.

BAYOU GUMBO

A Cajun treat from the bayou

½ C dry lima beans or 1 can　　2 C tomatoes, diced
　lima or butter beans*　　　　4 C vegetable stock
1 onion, chopped　　　　　　1 C fresh or frozen corn
1 green pepper, diced　　　　1½ C sliced okra
3 cloves (real cloves, not　　　1 t salt
　cloves of garlic)　　　　　　1¼ t allspice

Soak lima beans overnight in 2 C water (adding 1 t baking soda will reduce gas), drain and rinse.

Sauté the onion and green pepper with the cloves in water (or with some balsamic vinegar) until soft. Remove the cloves. Simmer all ingredients in a heavy covered pot for 5 hours or a slow cooker on high for 6 hours or on low for 8 to 10 hours. Prepare in the morning and come home to find dinner waiting for you.

This dish is tasty, but not spicy. Adding Tabasco or hot sauce will lend it an authentic Cajun tang.

Serve with brown rice and very low-fat corn bread, or a hearty whole wheat bread and a salad.

4 servings, each: Calories 124, Fat 1.2 g (8% CFF), Carbohydrate 25.3 g, Protein 5.9 g.

HEALTHY HEART HINT:

♥ To add a seafood flavor to your favorite dish, add a variety of sliced seaweeds. These can be found dried in most Asian markets.

---

*Cooking your own lima beans makes this a low-salt meal. Canned beans are high in sodium.

SPAGHETTI SQUASH AND ZUCCHINI CASSEROLE

Great for potlucks—you don't have to
bring home the serving dish

1 spaghetti squash
(2 to 2½ pounds)
1 C tomato sauce (or a 6-oz
can tomato paste + 4 T
water)
1 medium zucchini, grated
1 t finely chopped fresh
basil or ½ t dried basil
1 t dried oregano

1 t garlic powder
(or 2 cloves finely
chopped fresh garlic)
¼ t freshly ground black
pepper
¼ t salt (optional)
Serrano chili sauce or other
hot pepper (optional)

Preheat oven to 350°F. Cut spaghetti squash in half lengthwise. Carefully scrape out seeds without cutting into the squash. To microwave, place in a dish with ¼ C water, cover with plastic wrap and cook on high for 7 minutes. For stovetop, place half the squash cut-side down in a pot with 2 inches of water, cover and boil for 20 minutes. Squash is now half-cooked.

Scrape out squash with a fork to produce spaghetti-like strands. The thin hard shell will become a baking dish, so be careful not to puncture it. In a large bowl, add spaghetti squash strands, tomato sauce, grated zucchini and spices. Mix well and spoon into the shell (or a casserole dish), top with nutritional yeast, a little more garlic powder (and if desired, fat-free Parmesan substitute). Bake at 350°F for 25 minutes or until tender.

8 servings, each: Calories 95, Fat 0.186 g (1% CFF), Carbohydrate 22.95 g, Protein 3.66 g.

LENTILS AND RICE (DAAL BHAAT)

From the builders of the Taj Mahal

1 C brown lentils
2¾ C water
1 t black mustard seeds
1 t turmeric
1 t ground coriander
1 t ground cumin

1 small onion
2 cloves garlic
1 t fresh ginger
1 28-oz can of tomatoes
1 pot cooked brown rice

Boil lentils in water, then simmer for 40 minutes, or until the lentils are soft and water is absorbed. To microwave: decrease water to 1 C and and cook on high for about 5 minutes.

Heat mustard seeds and spices in a non-stick skillet, tightly covered until the black mustard seeds pop. Add the onions, garlic and ginger and cook until soft. Add the tomatoes with their liquid and cook until well blended. Add lentils, simmer for 2 minutes more. Serve over brown rice.

4 servings, each: Calories 316, Fat 1.79 g (5% CFF), Carbohydrate 63.67 g, Protein 10.97 g.

HEALTHY HEART HINT:

♥ Many recipes that call for beans can use lentils as a substitute. Lentils cook in only 30 minutes and are lower in fat than most beans. For each cup of lentils, add 2 C of water (onions, garlic and other spices can be added), bring to a boil and reduce heat to bubble slowly.

SHEPHERD'S PIE

An old English favorite

*1 lb potatoes (may use
 instant flakes)
1 14-oz can tomatoes
1½ oz TVP (textured
 vegetable protein)
 granules
½ t dried mixed herbs:
 basil, oregano, parsley,
 thyme, marjoram, etc.
 (optional)*

*½ t Worcestershire sauce
 (optional)
1½ lb root vegetables
 (such as leeks, turnips,
 carrots, etc)
3 oz tomato paste
½ cup non-fat Soy Moo
 or any low-fat soy or
 rice milk
4 T nutritional yeast flakes*

Preheat oven to 350°F. Peel potatoes and put on to boil (or use instant potato flakes). Empty tomatoes into a separate saucepan, add TVP. Bring to boil and reduce to simmer. Add herbs, Worcestershire sauce.

Cook vegetables lightly in separate pan. When vegetables are cooked, add to TVP mixture (add some cooking liquid if the TVP is too dry).

When potatoes are cooked, mash with soy or rice milk. Then sprinkle in the nutritional yeast flakes, and more milk if required. Stir until well mixed.

Place potatoes on top of the TVP and vegetable mix. Bake about 30 minutes. The potatoes should be slightly puffed up and browned on top. If not browned, put under the broiler for a few minutes.

4 servings, each: Calories 229, Fat 0.99 g (4% CFF), Carbohydrate 43.1 g, Protein 13.3 g.

SAVORY OATBURGERS

Make your own veggie burger for pennies

4 C water
*½ C salt-reduced soy sauce
    or tamari*
½ C nutritional yeast
1 large onion, diced
½ T garlic powder
*1 T each oregano and
    basil, dried*

1 t liquid smoke (optional)
*¼ C to 1 C mushrooms,
    fresh or canned
    (optional)*
*4 ½ C old-fashioned
    rolled oats*

In a medium pot, bring all ingredients except the oats to a boil. Turn heat to low and stir in oats. Cook for about 5 minutes, until the water is absorbed. Don't overcook. If too soupy, add some oats and cook for only a few more minutes until thickened.

Fill a rectangular non-stick baking pan with the mixture (makes square burgers—much easier than forming round patties). Use one large cookie sheet or two 12″ x 12″ pans to make patties about ½″ thick. (If patties are thinner, they'll dry out and be tough.)

Total cooking time is 45 minutes. Bake at 350°F for 25 minutes. Then use a utensil that won't scratch your pan to cut the giant burger into 3½″ to 4″ square burgers. Flip them over. Cook another 20 minutes. Serve on buns or as a main course, hot or cold. Can be frozen.

12 large burgers, each: Calories 147, Fat 1.98 g (12% CFF), Carbohydrate 25.1 g, Protein 7.9 g.

STUFFED SWEET PEPPERS

Full flavor without the meat

1 pot cooked brown rice	*1 t rosemary*
Low-salt tomato juice or	*1 t black pepper*
6-oz can tomato paste or	*2 cloves garlic, minced*
8-oz can tomato sauce	*(or 1 t garlic powder)*
4 T chopped dried onions	*2 T nutritional yeast*
2 16-oz cans chopped	*½ lb mushrooms*
(or stewed) tomatoes	*1 large onion*
1 t oregano	*Balsamic vinegar*
1 t thyme	*5-6 green bell peppers*

Prepare 3 C brown rice, but substitute half the water with tomato juice (or tomato paste or tomato sauce with the regular amount of water). Add 4 T of dried onions to the cooking liquid. When ready, set aside.

Pour 1½ cans of the tomatoes into a saucepan. Add all the spices and nutritional yeast, and simmer over low heat until ready to use.

Slice mushrooms and chop onions. Sauté both in a little balsamic vinegar until limp. Add mushrooms, onions and ½ can of tomatoes to the set-aside rice. Mix.

Clean peppers: cut top off each pepper and remove seeds and large veins. If peppers won't stand upright, slice a little off the bottom. Fill with rice mixture and set in a large oven pan. Pour tomato sauce over peppers, an inch or two deep in the pan.

Bake for 1 hour at 375°F, or until tender. Periodically baste peppers with the tomato sauce to keep them from drying out. Serve the tomato sauce from the pan as a side dish.

6 servings, each: Calories 538, Fat 4 g (7% CFF), Carbohydrate 113.9 g, Protein 13.5 g.

BEAN BURRITOS

Take these with you when you travel

1 can pinto beans
1 can black beans
1 can garbanzo beans
(chick-peas)
1 C roasted veggies (green
and red peppers, zucchini,
yellow squash, or any other)
2+ cloves of garlic

Salt-free seasoning
(Mrs. Dash)
Hot pepper to taste
Soft whole wheat tortillas or
baked corn taco shells
Shredded lettuce, tomato,
salsa and other burrito
trimmings

Combine all beans in saucepan and heat (if using fresh beans, soak overnight, then cook in 2 C water per cup of beans until soft). Cut up roasted veggies and add them along with garlic and seasoning to beans. Process or blend all ingredients together to the consistency you prefer— nearly whole beans, slightly lumpy, or creamy smooth. Simmer 20 minutes. Serve with lettuce, tomato, salsa, fat-free soy cheese and other trimmings, in soft tortillas (whole wheat or corn tortillas have less fat) or baked corn taco shells or toasted pita bread rounds.

You can use this bean recipe instead of meat for a taco filling and as a dip with fat-free corn chips.

6 servings, each: Calories 116, Fat 0.56 g (4% CFF), Carbohydrate 21.6 g, Protein 7.1 g.

HEALTHY HEART HINT:

♥ To make very low-fat taco shells, drape low-fat corn tortillas over two bars of an oven rack in an upside-down U and bake until crisp in a warm oven (325°F), about 10 to 15 minutes. Cool and stuff.

ROASTED EGGPLANT (MIRZA GHASSEMI)

A hint of India, but not too spicy

1 medium eggplant
1 medium onion, chopped
3 garlic cloves, minced
1 t mustard seed
1 t turmeric
1 dash cayenne (adjust to taste)

1 t curry powder
1 large tomato, peeled and seeded or ½ C canned tomatoes
¼ t black pepper
½ t salt

Roast the eggplants over a charcoal grill, or roast them in a 400°F oven until brown on the outside and soft on the inside. Cool and peel. Sauté the onions in water until translucent, then add garlic and mustard seed. Cook until the onions begin to turn golden. Stir in the turmeric, cayenne and curry. Add the eggplant pulp, onion mixture and tomato to a food processor and blend. Add half the tomato and taste. The more tomato you add, the sweeter it becomes. The traditional mixture is thick and red-brown. Add the salt and pepper. Serve over steamed brown rice.

3 servings, each: Calories 72.6, Fat 0.91 g (10% CFF), Carbohydrate 16.05 g, Protein 2.32 g.

HEALTHY HEART HINT:

♥ You can still use your barbecue. Many vegetables are delicious grilled, whether marinated or plain. While still hot, use the barbecue to cook sliced sweet potatoes, carrots and other veggies that you can refrigerate and use later as snacks.

SWEET POTATO AND GREEN BEANS DIABLO

A devilishly delightful combination

1 (9-oz) sweet potato, peeled,
cut into ¼"-lengthwise
strips
4 oz fresh green beans, tips
and strings removed

1 T Dijon mustard
1 T honey
¼ t cornstarch
⅛ t dried dill
Salt and pepper to taste

Light grill or preheat oven. Place sweet potato strips and green beans in center of a 14" x 14" sheet of heavy-duty aluminum foil. In small bowl, combine remaining ingredients; blend well. Drizzle over vegetables; stir gently to coat. Wrap with the aluminum foil, sealing securely with tight double folds. Place foil packet over medium heat or on charcoal grill 4 to 6 inches from flame (or medium-high heat on gas barbecue). Cook 20 to 25 minutes or until vegetables are crisp-tender. Open packet; stir gently. Serve immediately.

Oven option: Heat oven to 425°F. Prepare vegetables in foil packet as directed above. Bake for 35 to 40 minutes or until vegetables are crisp-tender. Open packet; stir gently.

4 servings, each: Calories 92.2, Fat 0.88 g (8% CFF), Carbohydrate 19.69 g, Protein 1.94 g.

HEALTHY HEART HINT:

♥ Sweet potatoes are not related to white potatoes. Persons with allergies to white potatoes can eat sweet potatoes or yams, which contain beta-carotene, an antioxidant known to fight cancer. For a snack treat, slice sweet potatoes, sprinkle with cinnamon or other spices, and bake in a medium oven until crispy.

ASPARAGUS AND SHIITAKE RISOTTO

East and West meet Cat Chow Mein Street

1 C dried shiitake mush-
rooms (or any dried
mushrooms)
1 C hot water
1 onion, chopped
1 T balsamic vinegar
2-4 cloves garlic, minced
8 sun-dried tomato slices,
not packed in oil
1½ T red wine, sherry or mirin
or ¼ C water

2 C rice (brown, white,
basmati or arborio)
4 C vegetable broth (or
Chick'n-Style Seasoning
and water)
½ lb asparagus, in
1-inch pieces
Salt and pepper to taste

Soak mushrooms in hot water for 15 minutes (keep under water and covered). Squeeze out excess water and cut into small pieces.

In a large pot, sauté onion in balsamic vinegar and a little water for a few minutes. Add garlic, diced sun-dried tomatoes and wine (or use ¼ C water). Cook until onion begins to brown. Add rice, stirring for about 1 minute. Add ½ C broth to deglaze pan. When broth boils, bring to medium heat and stir constantly. When broth is absorbed, add water in ½-cup increments, stirring constantly. After 10 minutes, add asparagus. Continue cooking until rice is tender, about 25 to 30 minutes. Season with salt and pepper. Serve immediately.

4 servings, each: Calories 546, Fat 3.25 g (5% CFF), Carbohydrate 85.24 g, Protein 20.53 g.

CAJUN-STYLE RED BEANS AND BROWN RICE

A Louisiana bayou tradition

1 lb dried pinto beans
2 C chopped yellow onions
1 C chopped green onions
1 C chopped green bell
    pepper
1 6-oz can tomato paste
1 t minced dried garlic
    (or 2 cloves chopped
    fresh garlic)
¾ t ground black pepper

½ t salt
¼ t oregano
¼ t thyme
1 T Worcestershire sauce
3 dashes Tabasco sauce
¼ t red cayenne pepper
    (optional; needed for
    Cajun flavor)
1 t celery flakes
6 C cooked brown rice

Wash beans and then soak for 12 hours. Drain water. Fill a large pot with beans; add water to ½" above beans' level. Add all remaining ingredients except the rice; cook over low heat 2 to 2½ hours, covered. Serve over cooked brown rice.

8 servings, each: Calories 431, Fat 2.21 g (4% CFF), Carbohydrate 85.24 g, Protein 20.53 g.

HEALTHY HEART HINT:

♥ Adding 1 T baking soda to the beans' soaking water will help reduce gas and discomfort. Do *not* cook beans with baking soda or salt added to the water.

COUSCOUS WITH SEVEN VEGETABLES (MOROCCAN STYLE)

A tasty meal from the Casbah

1 medium onion	*1 12-oz to 15-oz can*
3 C vegetable broth	*tomato sauce*
2 carrots, peeled	*¼ t cinnamon*
2 turnips, peeled	*½ t turmeric*
1 sweet potato	*¼ t curry powder*
1 zucchini	*Pinch of saffron threads*
1 red pepper	*(optional)*
1 can garbanzo beans,	*2 C couscous* (whole wheat*
drained	*or regular)*

In a large saucepan, sauté onion in a little broth until lightly browned. Add the remaining vegetable broth and bring to a boil. Cut all veggies into strips, julienne style. Transfer onion and broth to a large pot and add carrots, turnips and potato. Simmer 15 minutes. Lower heat and add zucchini and red pepper. Cook 20 minutes. Add beans, tomato sauce and spices. Cook until heated through.

In a separate pot, bring 2½ cups of water to a boil. Add couscous, cover and let stand 5 to 7 minutes away from heat. Fluff with a fork and serve with vegetable mix on top.

4 servings, each: Calories 746, Fat 4.55 g (5% CFF), Carbohydrate 155.4 g, Protein 27.72 g.

---

*Couscous is a pasta, like spaghetti, formed into small beads.

JAMAICAN BARLEY VEGETABLE CONFETTI

As interesting as reggae

1½ C uncooked barley
4½ C water
1 onion, coarsely chopped
2 cloves garlic, minced
1 small zucchini, quartered
lengthwise and then cut
into ¼" pieces

1 small red pepper, chopped
1 8-oz can mushrooms or
1 lb fresh, sliced
1 medium carrot, diced in
small pieces
1 C vegetable broth
*2 T Pickapeppa sauce**

In a medium size pot, boil the barley in 4½ C water for 45 minutes (or prepare according to package directions). Drain.

In a large pan, sauté the vegetables in vegetable broth for about 10 minutes, or until just tender. Add the Pickapeppa sauce and stir well. Stir in the cooked barley, mix well. Add more sauce if desired.

4 servings, each: Calories 418.4, Fat 4.1 g (8% CFF), Carbohydrate 88.25 g, Protein 17.45 g.

HEALTHY HEART HINT:

♥ Many of your favorite soups can be made into a main course by thickening them with a small amount of cornmeal, arrowroot or flour, and serving oven brown rice or pasta!

---

*Pickapeppa, the "ketchup" of Jamaica found on most every table, is a mix of toma-toes, vinegar, onions, mangoes, sugar, spices and peppers. It is more sweet than spicy. The 2 T in the recipe does not make it overly hot, but you may prefer to start with 1 T and then add more to your taste. Pickapeppa is available in local super-markets. If you can't find it, try 2 T A.1. steak sauce and a few dashes of Tabasco.

POCKET POTATO GORDITAS

From south of the border, this is quick and easy

4 potatoes, peeled and cubed	*1 clove garlic, minced*
1½ C water	*1 t green chili, canned or fresh*
1 t cumin	*1 bay leaf*
1 t oregano	*4 whole wheat pita*
1 t chili powder	*(pocket) breads*

Bring water to a boil. Reduce to medium high and add potatoes, spices, garlic and chilies. Stir occasionally to keep mixture from sticking to the bottom of the pot. After boiling for 8 to 10 minutes, reduce heat, cover and simmer about 20 minutes, or until it has thickened well.

Remove the bay leaf and fill the pita pockets with the mixture. Add salsa if desired. Gordita means "little fat one" in Spanish, so pack them round and full. These are just as delicious as leftovers.

4 servings, each: Calories 253, Fat 1.098 g (4% CFF), Carbohydrate 53.0 g, Protein 8.56 g.

HEALTHY HEART HINT:

♥ Pita bread can be used in place of tortillas or chapatis, or for a quick mini-pizza. You can substitute pita bread for sliced bread when making sandwiches, especially if you are traveling. Try whole wheat pita. Very low in fat, it can be cut into wedges and heated into crispy crackers in the oven.

SOUTH INDIAN LENTIL PANCAKES (ADAI)

Bring Bombay to your table

1 C mixed lentils (red, brown, green, etc.)	*2 C brown rice*
	½ t salt (optional)

The night before, wash and rinse the lentils thoroughly. When the rinse water runs clear, soak the lentils and rice together in a bowl with fresh water overnight. The next day, drain and grind into a semi-coarse paste in a blender, adding water as needed. Put the batter into a bowl, add salt, cover and let sit a few hours. This can be blended in the morning and will be ready to cook for dinner. For a sourdough flavor, let it ferment overnight.

Drop a ladleful of the batter in the center of a non-stick pan that is hot enough to make a drop of water dance. Push down in the center with a large spoon to make a thin, round pancake. When the top looks dry, wait 20 to 40 seconds more, turn and cook the other side. Serve immediately with a chutney (see the recipe for Cilantro Chutney). The batter can be refrigerated for about a week.

Add additional ingredients for variety. Try any combination of finely chopped onions, jalapenos, spinach, ginger, cumin seeds, garlic, curry powder, cinnamon or other favorite spices.

4 servings, each: Calories 445, Fat 2.3 g (5% CFF), Carbohydrate 89.95 g, Protein 15.29 g.

POTATO PASTA PIECES (*GNOCCHI*)

Marco Polo brought noodles from China,
but this is an original Italian dish

3 large baking potatoes
(about 2 lbs)
1 C whole wheat pastry
flour

½ t salt
3 T nutritional yeast
2 C low-fat *marinara or*
other pasta sauce

Microwave the potatoes in their skins for about 4 minutes
each or until tender (or steam or boil them). Drop them in
a bowl of cold water to cool, then peel and mash. Add flour,
salt and nutritional yeast, and mix well, kneading until
smooth. If the dough sticks, use a little flour. Form into rolls
about as round as a nickel. Cut into cube-size sections and
press each down lightly with a spoon or fork to make thinner in the middle.

Drop pasta pieces slowly into a 4-quart pot of boiling
water. When they rise to the top, take off heat and let sit 5
minutes. Drain and place pasta in a warm serving dish.
Cover with enough sauce to coat the pieces completely.
Serve with sauce on the side for those who prefer more.

Sweet potato can be substituted in the same proportion
to make a golden, slightly sweet pasta.

4 servings, each: Calories 271, Fat 0.92 g (2.2% CFF),
Carbohydrate 57.26 g, Protein 10.13 g.

HEALTHY HEART HINT:

♥ Most pasta is made from semolina, a white flour with
most of the fiber and vitamins removed. To get full nutrition
and fiber, use whole wheat or other whole grain pastas.

SEAFOOD-FLAVORED EGGPLANT

"Fruit of the Sea"—accent to an Oriental favorite

*1 large Japanese eggplant
or aubergine eggplant
4 scallions (green onions
can substitute), chopped
4 T low-salt soy sauce
3 T sugar
¼ C distilled white vinegar
3 T dry sherry (or mirin)*

*1 t crushed dried red pepper
6 slices ginger, size and
thickness of a quarter
1 strip (about 2" x 8") dashi-
kombu (dried kelp) or other
sea vegetable, diced finely
1 T cornstarch*

Cut stem end off eggplant. Slice Japanese eggplant into ¼" coins. If using aubergine (regular) eggplant, cut into thick slices and lightly salt both sides of eggplant. Set on paper towel for ½ hour. Dice eggplant into small cubes.

Separate white and green parts of scallions. In a small bowl, combine soy sauce, sugar and vinegar with ¼ cup of water. Heat 1 T dry sherry (or mirin—omit sugar if using) in a large skillet or wok. Add red peppers and stir. Add ginger, white part of scallions and sea vegetable. Stir-fry briefly until ginger becomes fragrant. Add eggplant and sauté approximately 8 to 10 minutes, stirring occasionally. If eggplant starts to stick, add a little water or wine. Add soy sauce mixture and cook over high heat until most of the liquid is evaporated and eggplant is thoroughly coated with reduced sauce—about 5 minutes. Combine 2 T sherry/mirin with cornstarch. Add chopped green part of scallions and sherry mixed with cornstarch. Stir and cook until thick. Serve hot over plain rice.

2 servings, each: Calories 172.6, Fat 0.35 g (5% CFF), Carbohydrate 37.03 g, Protein 5.26 g.

CABBAGE CASSEROLE

Stuffed cabbage, lasagna style

½ head cabbage
2 C cooked brown rice
½ C whole wheat couscous
¼ C raisins (optional)
½ C fresh or frozen corn
1 can chopped tomatoes
1 12-oz can tomato sauce
1 t fresh lemon juice

1 T brown sugar or brown
  rice syrup
¼ t each: cardamom,
  coriander, curry, pepper
  and garlic powder
Pinch allspice
⅛ t ground cloves (optional)

Slice cabbage diagonally. Pour hot water over it to make it limp. Drain. Mix rice, couscous, raisins and corn and set aside. Mix tomatoes with all other ingredients and spread 1 C in the bottom of a large ceramic casserole dish lightly coated with a one second non stick spray. Cover with layers of the cabbage and the rice mixture. Top with the rest of the tomato mixture and cover with foil. Bake at 325°F for 30 to 45 minutes, until bubbly. Serve hot with whole wheat bread and a salad.

This dish is similar to a savory stuffed cabbage, but the difficulties and disasters of stuffing have been avoided. For a fancier dish, the rice mixture can be rolled into cabbage leaves and skewered with a toothpick. Green peppers can be stuffed instead of using cabbage.

4 servings, each: Calories 567, Fat 3.79 g (5% CFF), Carbohydrate 10.02 g, Protein 15.98 g.

SPINACH AND MUSHROOM ROLL-UP PIE

A main course or gourmet hors d'oeuvre

Dough (or use 16-oz pkg. low-fat frozen bread dough):

1 C warm water (110°F)	*½ t sugar*
½ t salt	*3 C whole wheat pastry flour*
1 T yeast	*(can use bread flour)*

Put 1 C warm water in a large bowl; mix in ⅛ t salt, yeast and sugar. Let stand 5 minutes. Add flour and salt. Knead about 5 minutes. Roll into a smooth, elastic ball of dough. Cover and let rise until double in size, about 15 minutes. Punch down and roll into a rectangular shape.

Filling:

1 C TVP granules or flakes	*2 C mushrooms, sliced*
1 t salt	*10 oz frozen chopped spinach,*
1 t oregano	*thawed and drained*
1 t basil	*6 oz tomato paste*
1 t fennel seed	*2 oz soy milk or rice milk*
	for brushing top crust

Mix TVP in ½ C boiling water. Add salt, oregano, basil and fennel seed. In a large skillet, cook TVP mixture for a few minutes. Stir in mushrooms, spinach and tomato paste until heated through.

Preheat oven to 375°F. Spread filling evenly on top of dough and roll up like a jelly roll. Brush top with soy or rice milk. Bake 30 to 35 minutes. Check at 15 minutes; if crust begins to brown too much, cover with foil.

8 servings, each: Calories 277, Fat 1.50 g (5% CFF), Carbohydrate 42.03 g, Protein 29.13 g.

LONG RICE AND VEGETABLES ORIENTAL

Long rice is the Hawaiian name for rice noodles

¼ C mirin, sake or dry sherry
2 T ginger root, grated fresh
2 garlic cloves, minced
1 C carrots, thinly sliced
1 C broccoli stems, thinly sliced
1 C cabbage, thinly sliced
2 green onions
Optional: water chestnuts,
  bamboo shoots, pea pods
¼ C water
1 T hot pepper sauce or
  ½ t ground cayenne
  pepper (to taste)

1 T honey or brown rice
  syrup (omit if using
  mirin)
1 t Hoisin sauce (a Chinese
  sweet bean sauce found
  in Asian markets)
4 C rice noodles, cooked
  (according to package
  directions)
1 t to 3 T low-salt soy
  sauce (to taste)

Heat mirin (or sake or sherry) in a non-stick wok or skillet at medium heat until bubbling. Add ginger, garlic, carrots and broccoli. Stir-fry until carrots soften slightly, about five minutes. Add cabbage and green onions; cover and cook 3 minutes. Additional vegetables—water chestnuts, bamboo shoots, pea pods—may be added to taste. When cooked, remove vegetables to a separate dish.

Add water, ¼ of the pepper or hot sauce (later add more to taste), honey and Hoisin sauce to wok and heat until bubbling. Add noodles and stir-fry until thoroughly heated. Add vegetables and heat evenly. Add low-salt soy sauce.

8 servings, each: Calories 309, Fat 0.31 g (5% CFF), Carbohydrate 71.13 g, Protein 2.13 g.

"Instant" Tamale Pie

After a hard day's work, come home, spend five minutes preparing this, take a shower and enjoy a complete meal

1 can vegetarian non-fat
  chili and beans
1 C chunky salsa
1 C corn kernels (fresh
  cooked, frozen or canned)
1 C chopped steamed
  vegetables

2 C water
1 C + 1 T yellow stone-
  ground cornmeal
1 T freshly squeezed
  lemon juice
½ t mustard, Dijon style
½ t salt

Preheat oven to 350°F.

Mix chili, salsa, corn and vegetables, and pour into an 8″ x 8″ or 9″ x 7″ casserole.

In a quart saucepan, add 2 C boiling water to cornmeal, lemon juice, mustard and salt, and stir until mixed. On low heat, simmer, stirring continually until thickened. Add additional water if too thick to stir.

Spread cooked cornmeal mush over the vegetable/bean mixture. Bake for 30 minutes. Cool 10 minutes before serving.

4 servings, each: Calories 345, Fat 2.26 g (6% CFF), Carbohydrate 68.91 g, Protein 12.13 g.

(Nutritional analysis calculated with a 15-oz can Health Valley Spicy Vegetarian Chili with Black Beans and Pace salsa.)

PIMIENTO PASTA SAUCE

Tired of tomato-based sauces?
Here's a new taste treat

*2 large, ripe, sweet red bell
peppers (yellow peppers
can also be used)
2 T water (or 1 t balsamic
vinegar plus water)
to sauté
2 C onions, coarsely
chopped
2 t garlic, crushed
(3 cloves)*

*½ t red pepper flakes
(optional)
1 C vegetable stock
Salt and coarse freshly
ground black pepper
to taste
4 servings whole wheat
pasta (about 12 oz)
¼ C chopped fresh basil
(or 3 T dried basil)*

Clean peppers and remove seeds and inner ribs, then
chop coarsely. Heat sauté liquid in a large saucepan and
add peppers, cooking about 5 minutes, stirring and adding
more water if needed. Add onions, garlic and red pepper,
and continue cooking about 2 more minutes.

Add the stock, salt and pepper. Cover and simmer 15
minutes more. While sauce is simmering, cook pasta.

Remove sauce from heat and purée in a blender or food
processor. Return to pan, bring to boiling point and reduce
heat to simmer. Add basil and simmer about 3 more minutes.

4 servings, each: Calories 303.6, Fat 1.78 g (3% CFF),
Carbohydrate 70.87 g, Protein 15.47 g.

HEALTHY HEART HINT:

♥ Basil, oregano and parsley grow easily and well in a
window box at home. Many fresh herbs can be chopped
and frozen in zip-close bags. Spices retain their flavor longer
when stored air-sealed, away from light and heat.

POT STICKERS OR WON TON

An Oriental appetizer or soup treat—easy and quick

*8 oz vegetarian fat-free
   sausage*
*2 t fresh ginger root, grated
   (or 1 t powdered ginger)*
2 T salt-reduced soy sauce

*½ C cabbage, cooked and
   finely chopped*
*1 package frozen won ton
   wrappers (without egg)*

Defrost sausage a few patties at a time in the microwave, for about 30 seconds. Mix defrosted sausage, ginger, soy and cabbage. Lay out several won ton wrappers, then put a wad of the filling in the center of each wrapper (each sausage patty should make about 6 dumplings). Pinch the won ton wrappers closed at the top and hold together a moment.

These can be placed directly into a vegetable broth for won ton soup, or steamed to make pot stickers. After steaming they can be slightly browned in a non-stick pan to make "gyoza," which are dipped in a sauce of half vinegar and half soy sauce, with a little hot pepper optionally added.

To steam, place in a single layer in a steamer basket over boiling water for about 8 minutes.

Two brands of sausage that have worked well in this recipe are Garden Sausage (Wholesome & Hearty) and Gimme Lean Sausage Flavor (Lightlife).

About 24 dumplings, each: Calories 31.6, Fat 0.21 g (6% CFF), Carbohydrate 5.08 g, Protein 2.27 g.

STUFFED ONIONS FRANÇOIS

A naturally sweet surprise from the
Mediterranean countryside

6 large Maui or Vidalia
  onions (if not found,
  use yellow onions)
1 C mushrooms, chopped
3 cloves garlic, crushed
1 apple, peeled, cored,
  chopped (1 C)
2 T fresh parsley, minced

2 T fresh marjoram, minced
  (or 1 t dried)
1 t lemon juice
¼ t paprika
Salt and pepper to taste
1 C cooked wild rice
1 C vegetable stock

Preheat oven to 400°F. Cut ¼ inch off top and bottom of onions, peel off dry layers. Bake onions, root end down, in baking dish for 30 minutes, or until golden brown. Let cool and hollow out each onion from top, leaving ½-inch shell (outer most 2 to 4 layers).

Chop 1 C of reserved onion and sauté with mushrooms in a medium hot pan until onions are transparent. Add garlic and apple and continue cooking 3 minutes. Add parsley, marjoram, lemon juice, paprika, salt and pepper; combine the sautéed mixture with the cooked rice.

Fill each onion shell with rice mixture. Pour enough stock to cover bottom of onions (about ½ inch). Bake for 20 minutes, basting the stuffed onions with stock occasionally.

One serving per onion, each: Calories 180, Fat 1.08 g (5% CFF), Carbohydrate 38.24 g, Protein 5.76 g.

HEALTHY HEART HINT:

♥ Onions can be baked the day before and refrigerated, to be stuffed and final baked just before serving.

PAELLA JARDINERA

This Spanish favorite is typically packed with seafood.
The traditional flavor is captured with the sea
vegetable/kelp, but it is optional

2 cloves garlic, crushed
1 large onion, sliced
4 celery stalks, sliced
1 t paprika
1 each red, green and
yellow bell pepper, cored,
seeded and cut into
squares or strips
1 C whole green beans
2 C long grain or basmati
brown rice
14-oz can peeled tomatoes
2 pinches saffron strands
(real Spanish saffron seems
expensive, but less than 75
cents worth is used here)

1 large piece dashi-kombu
sea vegetable (½-oz), cut
into ½" squares
(optional)
4 C vegetable stock
14-oz can artichoke hearts
(be sure they are not in
oil), *drained and halved*
1 C frozen peas
1 T lemon juice
2 T chopped parsley
Salt and pepper to taste
Lemon wedges and
parsley to garnish

Sauté garlic, onion and celery until onion is transparent.
Add paprika, bell peppers and beans and sauté for 2 to 3
minutes. Add rice and cook for 2 minutes, stirring constantly. Add tomatoes with their juice, saffron, kombu and
stock and simmer gently for 20 minutes, stirring frequently,
until almost all liquid has been absorbed. If rice isn't tender,
cover and simmer 5 minutes longer. Add remaining ingredients (except garnish) and heat gently for about 5 minutes.
Garnish with lemon wedges and parsley to serve.

4 servings, each: Calories 375.5, Fat 2.98 g (7% CFF),
Carbohydrate 74.32 g, Protein 14.21 g.

MAHARAJA RICE

A mild yet exotic pilaf

*1 C brown rice, preferably
basmati or long grain
1 medium onion, chopped
2 T vegetable stock (may
use water, soy sauce or
dry wine to sauté)*

*4 cloves
1 small stick cinnamon
3 bay leaves
1 clove garlic (minced)
12-oz package frozen peas*

Rinse rice until water is clear and allow to soak 30 minutes in cold water. Sauté onions in stock on medium heat, until they start to become transparent. Add cloves, cinnamon, bay leaves and garlic; stir. Add rice and stir until rice starts to become slightly golden. Add 2 C cold water and allow pot to come to a boil. Add peas; stir. Lower heat and simmer covered until the rice is cooked. Let stand uncovered until extra water evaporates.

To prepare using an automatic rice cooker, follow the directions above, add all ingredients including peas to 2 C water in rice cooker. Mix well.

4 servings, each: Calories 430.4, Fat 2.96 g (6% CFF), Carbohydrate 88.49 g, Protein 12.24 g.

HEALTHY HEART HINT:

♥ Leftover rice or pasta can be frozen and quickly microwaved for later use. Put single servings in zip-close sandwich bags, seal all but one corner and then squeeze the air out from the bottom up, sealing completely when all the air is out. This will keep frozen indefinitely.

CREAMED LEEK AND POTATO BAKE

A heart-safe way to make a hearty Welsh favorite

2 large leeks, chopped
1 red bell pepper, diced
3 whole wheat matzos,
  broken (or the equivalent
  of any fat-free wheat
  cracker)
1 C hot water
6 oz low-fat *soy milk or*
  rice milk

5 large mushrooms, sliced
4 medium potatoes,
  microwaved, baked or
  boiled, peeled and sliced
3 T nutritional yeast
1 T minced chives for top

Preheat oven to 350°F. Sauté leeks in a non-stick skillet in a little water, covered, until soft. Add red pepper and sauté 5 minutes more. Combine matzos with water in bowl, soak 3 minutes or until soft. Drain, squeeze out excess water. Combine leek mixture and matzos with remaining ingredients, except yeast and chives. Stir until fully mixed. Pour into a non-stick shallow 2-qt. casserole. Sprinkle yeast over top, followed by chives. Bake 35 to 40 minutes, until top is slightly browned. Let stand 10 minutes, cut and serve.

As a main vegetable dish, this is rich and filling. By adding vegetable stock or water and then blending, this becomes a nutritious and thick cold-weather soup.

8 servings, each: 179.1 Calories, Fat 0.84 g (4% CFF), Carbohydrate 39.93 g, Protein 6.49 g.

LASAGNA ROMANA

You'll swear it was packed with cheese

2 onions, chopped
2 carrots, grated
½ C red wine
3 cloves garlic or 4 t crushed garlic
1 box (8 oz) mushrooms
2 cans Italian-style stewed tomatoes
2 8-oz cans tomato sauce
2 T basil
1 t oregano
¼ t cayenne pepper

1 T Italian seasoning
1 lb lite firm tofu (1½ boxes)
1 T Salad Sprinkle*
¼ C parsley, chopped
2 T low-salt soy sauce
1 box (12 oz) whole wheat lasagna pasta
1 box (10 oz) frozen spinach, thawed and chopped
Low-fat soy parmesan substitute (optional)

In a large skillet, braise onions and carrots in ½ C wine for 5 minutes. Add garlic and mushrooms; cook until the mushrooms are soft. Add stewed tomatoes and tomato sauce, basil, oregano, cayenne pepper and Italian seasoning. Mash tofu, add Salad Sprinkle, parsley and soy sauce, and mix. Be sure to use lite tofu—regular tofu will more than double the fat.

Preheat oven to 350°F. It is not necessary to precook lasagna pasta; just cover it with cold water for 10 minutes and pat dry. Pasta will absorb juices and cook fully in casserole.

In large baking dish, layer with enough sauce to cover bottom, add layers of lasagna pasta, then tofu mix, then chopped spinach, and repeat until all ingredients are used.

Bake 45 minutes at 350°F. Serve.

6 servings, each: Calories 318.7, Fat 2.77 g (7% CFF), Carbohydrate 62.26 g, Protein 19.34 g.

---

*Saltless Salad Sprinkle, a combination of dried vegetables and spices—red pepper, black pepper, lemon peel, celery, chervil, green onion, green bell peppers—is available in many supermarkets.

EGGPLANT PARMIGIANA

An authentic Italian tradition without the fat

1 large eggplant, sliced
4 T EnerG egg replacer
plus 8 T water, whipped
to peaks
1 C Corn Flakes, crushed,
with 1 t each garlic
powder, onion powder,
Italian seasoning

8 oz whole wheat pasta
2 C fat-free spaghetti sauce
12 oz fat-free soy
mozzarella cheese
4 t low-fat soy parmesan
cheese

Slice eggplant in ½" thicknesses, dip in whipped egg replacer and then in Corn Flakes mixture. Place slices on non-stick cookie sheet and bake at 350°F for 30 minutes or until tender.

While eggplant is cooking, boil pasta in 2 quarts of water until done. Rinse in cold water.

When eggplant is done, remove and place ⅓ of the spaghetti sauce on the bottom of the sheet, then the layer of eggplant, another ⅓ of spaghetti sauce and a layer of thinly sliced soy mozzarella, sprinkled with the soy parmesan. Reduce oven to 275°F and bake 15 minutes more.

Put the remaining spaghetti sauce on the pasta and serve with toasted garlic bagels and a salad.

4 servings, each: Calories 424, Fat 1.59 g (3% CFF), Carbohydrate 67.83 g, Protein 39.89 g.

GINGER BOK CHOY

Can be served cold as a salad or as a hot dish

*1 lb bok choy (Chinese
    cabbage)
1 T white vinegar
1 t sugar
1 t Dijon mustard*

*2 t low-salt soy sauce
1 clove garlic, finely
    chopped
1 T fresh ginger, finely
    chopped or grated*

Rinse bok choy leaves under cool water to clean. Bok choy can be microwaved in a covered dish (no added liquid) for about 5 minutes, or steamed until tender or stalks begin to turn translucent and are soft.

Combine vinegar, sugar, mustard, soy, garlic and ginger, and mix well. Warm to blend flavors.

To serve cold as a salad, dip bok choy into very cold water until crisp. Drain and refrigerate. Refrigerate sauce until cool; spoon over bok choy at the table.

To serve hot, chop bok choy into bite-size pieces. Cover with sauce and serve with brown rice or rice noodles.

4 servings, each: Calories 25.6, Fat 0.28 g (10% CFF), Carbohydrate 3.52 g, Protein 2.27 g.

HEALTHY HEART HINT:

♥ Many dishes that call for cabbage can be made with vegetable greens. Use the stems and leaves of mustard, collards, carrot and other greens.

YAMPLE CASSEROLE

Enjoy a festive holiday treat at any time of year

*2 large yams or sweet
   potatoes
2 firm apples, peeled, cored
   and cut into thin slices
1 package frozen corn or
   1 can (12-oz) corn,
   drained*

*8 oz fat-free vegetarian
   sausage
½ t cinnamon
¼ t nutmeg*

Peel sweet potatoes or yams and cut into ½"-thick slices. Boil the sweet potato slices until almost tender.

Mix all ingredients together and spoon into a covered ceramic baking dish. Bake at 350°F until the apples are tender, about 45 minutes. Serve hot.

4 servings, each: Calories 210.4, Fat 0.41 g (2% CFF), Carbohydrate 40.36 g, Protein 11.33 g.

1 C of your favorite green vegetables (broccoli, zucchini, long eggplant, kale, collard or mustard greens, spinach, etc.) can be added to this casserole to make a one-dish meal.

HEALTHY HEART HINT:

♥ If you don't care for yams or sweet potatoes, many yam dishes can be made with pumpkin or other winter squashes.

TREATS

DELUXE CORN BREAD

Easy to microwave or oven bake, and very low-fat

1 T EnerG egg replacer
with 4 T water
1 C low-fat soy milk or
rice milk
½ C fresh or frozen corn
kernels
1¼ C whole wheat or
unbleached bread flour

¾ C corn meal (yellow
or white)
⅛ C sugar or honey (or
fruit-based sweetener)
2 t baking powder
½ t salt
Optional spicy version:
add chili peppers or
hot sauce to taste

Preheat oven to 400°F. Whip egg replacer with water and add wet ingredients (milk, corn, and honey or fruit, if using). In a separate bowl, mix the dry ingredients well. Add dry to wet and stir *gently* until evenly distributed, but don't over-mix. Pour in a non-stick pan (bread-loaf or 8" x 8") and bake for 20 to 25 minutes. (When a knife blade comes out clean, it's done.)

Microwave directions: As above, mix wet, mix dry, combine until moistened. Pour batter into a non-stick 9" microwave-safe pie plate or round cake pan. Cook on high for 5 to 6 minutes or until the surface appears dry. Rotate after 2 minutes. Let stand 5 minutes before serving.

6 servings, each: Calories 205, Fat .898 g (4% CFF), Carbohydrate 44.9 g, Protein 5.79 g.

HEALTHY HEART HINT:

♥ When using egg replacer for baked goods, whip the powder with water until foamy. When mixing later with other ingredients, mix only until just evenly blended, or results will be dense and flat.

BETTER UN-BUTTER BROWNIES

A chocolate lover's delight

Dry: ½ *C whole wheat flour*   *1 t baking powder*
       ⅓ *C cocoa*   ¼ *t salt*

Wet: 1 *T EnerG egg replacer*   ⅔ *C sugar*
         with 4 T water   1 *t vanilla*
       ½ *C puréed prunes or*
       plums (one 4-oz jar of
       unsweetened baby food
       prunes or plums)

In one bowl, mix egg replacer with water and add the other wet ingredients. In another bowl, mix the dry ingredients well and then add to the wet. Mix only until evenly blended. Over-mixing will cause the brownies to be flat (and chewy). Bake in a non-stick pan at 350°F for 20 to 25 minutes or until edges look dry and start to pull away from the pan. Can also be microwaved on high for 6 minutes.

8 servings, each: Calories 115, Fat .803g (6% CFF), Carbohydrate 25.65 g, Protein 2.51 g.

HEALTHY HEART HINT:

♥ Use non-stick pans or spray a regular pan with one second's worth of Pam (or other non-stick spray). These sprays contain a form of fat, so use sparingly. Instead of trying to coat the pan with spray, use a small amount in the center and then spread it with a folded paper towel. Do *not* use oil to "grease" a pan; even a little oil adds extra fat that is not required.

BUCKWHEAT PANCAKES (OR WAFFLES)

For breakfast or dessert

Dry:

1 C buckwheat flour
1 C whole wheat flour
1 t cinnamon
1 T baking powder
1 T EnerG egg replacer
½ C raisins (optional)

Wet:

1 t vanilla
1 C water
¼ C unsweetened
   applesauce (optional)

Combine dry ingredients and vanilla. Add water and applesauce (if desired) and mix gently until blended with most (but not all) lumps gone. Do not over-mix. Add water to thin the batter if needed.

Heat a non-stick griddle or pan to about 350°F (or until a drop of water dances on the surface). Spray with a small amount of Pam (or other cooking spray), using a paper towel corner to wipe it evenly on the entire cooking surface. Spoon batter onto griddle. Turn the pancakes when no more bubbles appear on top or when slightly brown on bottom.

Pancakes are a challenge to creativity. Raisins, berries and diced fruit can be added to the batter. Coconut flavor and many extracts (banana, almond, mint, etc.) will yield new and interesting treats. Non-fat chocolate or carob chips give a cookie-like treat for kids (of all ages).

8 pancakes, each: Calories 114, Fat 0.76 g (6% CFF), Carbohydrate 24.5 g, Protein 3.9 g.

OATMEAL COOKIES

America's favorite—full of fiber, but very low in fat

1 C mashed bananas
1 C confectioners' (finely
* powdered) sugar*
1 C brown sugar
1 T EnerG egg replacer +
* ¼ cup water*
1 t vanilla
½ t salt
1 t baking soda

2 C whole wheat pastry
* flour*
2½ C oats, rolled or steel
* cut, or for oatmeal*
2 or 3 C raisins, dates,
* chocolate chips, carob*
* chips, dried fruit in any*
* combination*

Thoroughly blend bananas and sugars with a hand or electric mixer. Add egg replacer and water and beat thoroughly. Blend in vanilla, salt, baking soda, flour and oats, beating at medium speed after each addition. Stir in other ingredients. Press golf-ball size scoops onto a non-stick baking sheet 2″ apart. Bake at 400°F for 8 to 10 minutes or until brown. Allow time to cool completely. Makes about 2 dozen cookies, depending on size.

Per cookie: Calories 155, Fat 1.2 g (7% CFF), Carbohydrate 35.1 g, Protein 3.24 g.

GRAPE-NUTS™ BARS

Keep some with you for a low-fat snack

3 C Grape-Nuts cereal
1 C non-fat Soy Moo, or
   any low-fat soy milk or
   rice milk

1 C unsweetened applesauce
1 C raisins
2 t vanilla extract

Preheat oven to 350°F. Mix all ingredients together. Pour into a non-stick 9" x 9" baking dish. Bake for 35 minutes or until firm. Cool and cut into 12 squares.

To add some interesting or favorite taste variations, add 1 t or more of cocoa powder or any flavor extract, such as coconut, banana, almond, mint. Various spices may also be added: nutmeg, allspice, cinnamon, ginger, clove, lemon and orange peel.

These bars keep well in the freezer and are excellent for traveling. With 1% or lite low-fat soy milk, these are still only 4% CFF, and with regular soy milk, only 6% CFF.

12 squares, each: Calories 164, Fat 0.41 g (2% CFF), Carbohydrate 37.7 g, Protein 4.7 g.

HEALTHY HEART HINT:

♥ Soy milk is not necessarily low-fat. Regular soy milk has 5 g fat from 150 calories per 8 oz serving, or 30% calories from fat. Lite soy milk and rice milk have 3 g of fat in 150 calories per serving—18% CFF. Health Valley Soy Moo has 110 calories, zero fat.

CHOCOLATE PUDDING CAKE

Something to never make when you're home alone

1 C flour (try ½ C whole
    wheat mixed with
    ½ C white)
⅔ C sugar
2 T cocoa
2 t baking powder
⅛ t salt

½ C water
2 T applesauce
1 t vanilla
⅔ C brown sugar
¼ C cocoa
1¾ C hot water

Mix the first eight ingredients together. Spray 8" x 8" baking pan for 1 second with non-stick cooking spray (Pam), spread with paper towel, and then pour in mixture. Mix brown sugar and cocoa and sprinkle over the batter. Pour the hot water over the entire top surface. Bake at 350°F for about 45 minutes.

The topping sinks through the cake to form a pudding layer at the bottom. This cake tastes so rich it's hard to believe there are no fat or eggs in it. Most people prefer it chilled, but it can be served at room temperature or even warm (if you can't wait). It will keep for several days, but do not freeze or the pudding will turn watery.

6 servings, each: Calories 314.8, Fat 0.69 g (2% CFF), Carbohydrate 76.3 g, Protein 4.65 g.

HEALTHY HEART HINT:

♥ Cocoa powder is very low in fat compared to regular or baker's chocolate. For a chocolate topping, mix cocoa powder and sugar with just enough water to thicken and mix over heat.

QUICK RICE PUDDING

An old-fashioned favorite for your left-over cooked rice

3 C cooked brown rice
4 C vanilla flavored non-
fat soy milk (Soy Moo)
1 C pitted chopped dates
or date pieces

¾ C raisins or currants
½ t nutmeg
1 t vanilla extract

In a large, heavy saucepan, add all ingredients except nutmeg and vanilla. Bring to a boil and immediately reduce to a simmer, stirring constantly for 10 minutes. Remove from heat and add nutmeg and vanilla; stir. Serve warm or chilled. Dates will blend into the pudding, which will be thick and smooth.

6 servings, each: Calories 361.8, Fat 1.12 g (3% CFF), Carbohydrate 83.86 g, Protein 8.70 g.

For an extra treat, add ¼ C "craisins"—dried sweetened cranberries—instead of one-third of the raisins. A sprinkle of cinnamon also adds a new flavor.

HEALTHY HEART HINT:

♥ To sweeten dessert dishes, add a small amount of pure maple sugar. A little goes a long way.

ICE DREAM

Ever wonder what to do with those over-ripe bananas?
Try this non-dairy, no-sugar dessert, as
rich and creamy as ice cream

4 frozen bananas
8 oz of your favorite fresh or frozen fruit

When bananas turn black or are too ripe to eat, peel and enclose each in plastic wrap and then freeze. Using a blender, mix frozen bananas and fruit until smooth. Strawberries overwhelm the banana flavor and taste like strawberry ice cream. Other fruits, especially sweeter ones, often are improved by adding 1 t of lemon or lime juice.

4 servings, each: 185.1 Calories, Fat 0.89 g (4% CFF), Carbohydrate 41.64 g, Protein 2.49 g.

(Nutritional analysis for 4 bananas and 8 oz. fresh strawberries.)

HEALTHY HEART HINT:

♥ To make ice cream pie, blend 1 C Grape-Nuts with ½ C frozen apple juice concentrate, press into a pie pan and fill with Ice Dream. Freeze 3 hours before serving.

An Introduction
to Some Less
Well-Known Foods

Until you become familiar with the many new and delicious foods that so many people have never heard of, this short glossary of some of them should help you get started.

ADZUKI BEANS Low in fat and easily digestible, high in protein. These small, dark red beans are used in sweetcakes and puddings. Also known as aduki or azuki beans.

AGAR A gelatin substitute produced from sea vegetables, used for preparing dressings, gelatin type salads and desserts, puddings and pie fillings. Available in flakes or in foam-like solid cubes The cubes are much more economical, the flakes more convenient. One tablespoon of flakes is dissolved in about one cup of liquid and boiled. Use only after dissolving—agar thickens gradually but effectively.

AMARANTH An ancient Aztec staple, the seeds vary in color from dark purple to yellow. Rich in lysine, an amino acid not common in most grains, amaranth is high in protein, calcium, phosphorous and fiber.

AMAZAKE A traditional Japanese ingredient made by mixing koji, a cultured grain, with cooked sweet rice and then fermenting. Used as a sweetener and leavener for baked goods and for making creamy dairy-free puddings, pie fillings or malt-like beverages. Available in different flavors.

ARAME Brown seaweed usually dried into dark, wiry threads, with a mild, slightly sweet flavor. After soaking in water about 5 minutes, it becomes twice its size. High in minerals, vitamins and protein, especially calcium and potassium. Used in soups, stir-fries, salads and vegetable dishes.

ARROWROOT A thickener for shiny, transparent sauces. Dissolve in cold water and add at the end of cooking, as arrowroot-thickened sauces tend to break down if cooked too long. It can be substituted for cornstarch in equal amounts.

ARUGULA A spicy salad green, also called roquette or rocket. Mostly seen in western Asia and the Middle East. A member of the mustard family, it has dark green narrow leaves with deep lobes.

BAKING POWDER A mixture of alkali (usually baking soda) and acid that releases carbon dioxide gas when moistened to make baked goods rise without yeast. Most prepared baking powders become neutralized quickly on the shelf and fail to yield good results. Mixing equal parts of baking soda and cream of tartar (tartaric acid) at the time of use will give better results.

BALSAMIC VINEGAR This aromatic, somewhat syrupy Italian vinegar is made from grapes, and tastes more like a sweet wine than vinegar. Aging in balsam-wood casks gives it a dark amber color and its name. Used as a seasoning and in dressings and marinades. Popular varieties cost less than $10 for a 20-oz bottle, but true, aged balsamic vinegar can cost over $100 for a 25 ml (one cup) bottle.

BARLEY MALT SYRUP Made from sprouted, dried barley, it is about half as sweet as refined sugar and is more evenly metabolized than cane or beet sugar. A dark and thick natural sweetener, use as a substitute for honey or molasses or in baked goods.

BASMATI RICE An aromatic long-grain rice with a light flavor, native to India and Pakistan but now grown in the U.S. It increases in length when cooked, giving a light, fluffy, sweet-smelling rice.

BLACKSTRAP MOLASSES From the "bottom of the barrel" in making sugar, it contains very high amounts of many essential nutrients, including calcium, iron, potassium and phosphorous. With its stronger taste, use half as much in recipes calling for regular molasses.

BROWN RICE SYRUP A natural sweetener prepared by adding dried sprouted barley or barley enzymes to cooked rice, then fermenting the mixture until the rice starch breaks down to sugars. Like barley malt syrup, brown rice syrup is moderately sweet, and its sugars are absorbed gradually by the body rather than producing a sudden sugar "high."

BULGUR This is wheat that has been precooked, dried and cracked. This light, nutty-tasting Middle Eastern grain is available in various consistencies, from coarse to fine. Place in boiling water and simmer a few minutes to prepare.

CAROB These pods of the locust tree, dried, roasted and ground, have a flavor similar to chocolate. John the Baptist is said to have survived in the wilderness on carob, sometimes called St. John's Bread.

CHUTNEY Sweet, tart and sometimes hot relishes made of fruits, vegetables, spices and herbs, they can vary greatly. Used as a condiment for East Indian, Southeast Asian and Mediterranean dishes.

COUSCOUS Small pieces of pasta, couscous is precooked and is ready after 5 to 10 minutes of soaking. A North African starch staple used in almost any kind of dish.

CURRY POWDER A blend of various spices, differing greatly by region. May contain coriander, fenugreek, cumin, cayenne or other chili peppers, black pepper, cardamom, mustard seed, onion powder, ginger, clove, garlic, bay leaves, nutmeg, cinnamon, poppy seeds, mace, celery, salt and often turmeric (which is used for color as well as flavor). The leaf of the curry plant may be used in preparing the spice, possibly giving it its name.

DAIKON A member of the cabbage family, daikon is an icicle-shaped, bulbous white radish from the Far East. Sweet when cooked, it has a bite when used raw. Available fresh, dried or pickled.

DULSE A slightly salty, nutty-tasting, reddish-purple sea vegetable. Dulse is toasted for snacks, shredded raw for salads, or sautéed. Rich in iron, potassium and magnesium.

EGG REPLACER For leavening and binding baked goods that usually call for eggs. Made from food starches, it has no preservatives, artificial flavorings, sugar, sodium or cholesterol. It can be whipped for merengue or used in powder form instead of whole eggs or egg whites. The most common brand is *EnerG,* in a yellow box.

FENNEL A bulb topped by celery-like stalks and fine feathery leaves. Used in Mexican and Italian cuisine, it has a slightly sweet licorice taste when raw and a more subtle taste when cooked.

GLUTEN Made by eliminating the starch and bran from wheat flour, which is then kneaded and simmered in flavored broth. It is found in rice, kamut, barley, oats, rye and triticale and spelt. Gluten flour is often added to low-gluten bread dough to make it rise more. Cooked to look and taste like meat and fish of almost every kind. Used as meat in stews, stir-fries and sandwiches. Now available in quick-cooking varieties and fully prepared, often difficult to tell from ham, chicken, beef and many other flavors. Called seitan (in Japan) and kofu (in China).

HERBES DE PROVENCE A bouquet of southern French herbs usually containing marjoram, oregano, savory, rosemary, thyme, lavender leaves and fennel seeds, all dried or fresh.

JICAMA A large turnip-shaped root vegetable, with crisp and slightly sweet white flesh beneath a rough-textured light brown skin. Retains a crunchy texture when cooked. Low calorie and low sodium, it is high in potassium. Often eaten raw with citrus juice.

KASHA Hulled, toasted buckwheat groats. Tan-colored raw groats become reddish-brown when toasted. Quick-cooking kasha is high in protein, iron, calcium and B-vitamins.

KELP The largest marine plants, with nearly 1,000 species. Sold in powdered form or sheets, kelp is a nutritious and flavorful salt substitute, rich in calcium and iodine. It is said to help cleanse the body of toxins and radioactive matter.

KOMBU A sea vegetable (kelp), usually sold in dried dark-green strips. It contains glutamic acid, a natural flavor-enhancer and tenderizer, but it does not usually cause the same reaction as monosodium glutamate (MSG).

KUDZU A powdered dried root of a vine used as a thickening and gelling agent for sauces, puddings and pie fillings. A tasteless and odorless white starch, it is dissolved in cold water before adding to hot liquids.

LEGUMES A nutritious family of plants that includes peas, beans, lentils, clover and alfalfa. Legumes nourish themselves by creating nitrogen-rich soil.

LENTIL A convex (lens-shaped) seed of a legume. Low in fat and quicker cooking than beans, lentils can be used in similar ways as beans.

LIQUID SMOKE Distilled from wood smoke, just a few drops of this clear, non alcoholic liquid can give a deep smokey flavor and aroma.

MIRIN Sweetened rice wine for cooking Japanese dishes. Brewed from sweet brown rice, rice koji and water. Used in sauces, marinades, dressings and glazes, and in vegetable and noodle dishes.

MISO Fermented soybean paste; may have other grains or beans added. Darker misos are usually aged longer and are saltier. Used in sauces, soups, stews, beans, salad dressings and spreads.

MUNG BEANS Small green or yellow spherical beans, from the same family as kidney beans. Often used as sprouts. When peeled and split, they are yellow. In India they are known as *mung dahl*.

NORI A seaweed dried and pressed into papery sheets. When toasted, turns dark green to brown. Rich in vitamin A and protein, it emulsifies fat and helps break down cholesterol. Used as a wrapper for sushi, grains and vegetables. Used in small flakes as a garnish for stir-fries, soups and salads, and as a teriyaki-flavored snack. Also called laver.

NUTRITIONAL YEAST A killed yeast product, it cannot be used to make bread rise or ferment beer. Usually a yellow powder or flakes. Sometimes called brewer's yeast because it can be derived from byproducts of beer-making. Adds a light cheese-like flavor to many dishes; it is rich in many minerals and some vitamins. Some makers enrich it with vitamin B_{12}, the preferred choice.

PITA BREAD A Middle Eastern flat, round bread that can be opened and stuffed with fillings. Usually made without oil, it is often available in whole wheat and flavored varieties. Also called pocket bread.

POLENTA A thick mush of cornmeal. Can be made with a special corn flour or bought ready-made. It can be boiled, baked or grilled.

QUINOA Grain-like plant that is higher in protein than grains, with balanced proportions of all eight essential amino acids. The bitter-tasting saponins, a natural protective resin, can be easily rinsed off. Quinoa enlarges nearly five times during cooking. Used as any grain or in salads.

RICE VINEGAR Made from fermented rice or sake (rice wine). Flavor is enhanced and color turns golden with aging.

SAKE Rice wine common in Japan. Used to flavor sauces, marinades and dressings.

SEA SALT Containing trace elements that are processed out of regular table salt, it is made by evaporating unpolluted sea water. Usually sea salt is sold without aluminum-based anti-caking agents, which have been linked to the onset of Alzheimer's disease.

SEITAN See *gluten*.

SHIITAKE Large oriental mushrooms, fresh or dried, valued for their rich flavor and nutritional content, and reported to strengthen the immune system. Small amounts add a distinctive flavor to stews, soups, sauces, stir-fries, and noodle and grain dishes.

SHOYU Brewed, aged sauce made from soybeans, wheat, water and salt (often more than 1,000 mg per tablespoon). Adding it near the end of cooking preserves its flavor. Often available in reduced-salt varieties. (See **TAMARI**).

SOBA Noodles made of all buckwheat flour or a combination of buckwheat and wheat flours. May also contain wild yam *(jinenjo)*, mugwort, lotus root, green tea or other ingredients.

TAHINI Sesame seed paste made from roasted or hulled raw seeds. It is sesame oil (more than 80 percent calories from fat) with seed hulls.

TAMARI Wheat-free soy sauce made from soybeans, salt and water. Stronger flavor than shoyu, can be added earlier in cooking. As with shoyu, very high sodium content; available in reduced-salt varieties.

TEMPEH Hulled, split, cooked and fermented soybeans formed into cakes. Can also be made from grains, lentils or other beans. An Indonesian staple.

TOFU Bean curd cake. Tofu is made by coagulating soymilk with a mineral (usually calcium), draining off the whey and pressing. Tofu can be mashed, blended, marinated, simmered, steamed, baked, broiled or sautéed. Storing refrigerated in a covered container in water that is changed daily will allow it to last up to a week after opening. Freezing overnight will give it a crumbly, ricotta cheese texture. Varies from 40 percent to 60 percent calories from fat. Lite tofu, 28 percent calories from fat (labeled "1%"), is recommended.

TOMATILLO A small, tart, lemony flavored tomato-like fruit, with a yellow-green to purple color. Best bought in its brown husk, which is removed before cooking. Tends to thicken sauces.

TURMERIC An Indian herb used for coloring (bright yellow to dark orange) and flavoring. Often seen in curry and East Indian dishes, small amounts can color without adding a distinctive flavor. Also called bloodroot and goldenseal—these are related but are not true turmeric.

UDON Japanese linguini-like rice or wheat noodles.

UMEBOSHI Japanese pickled plums. Available also as a paste and "vinegar" (the pickling brine).

WAKAME Dark kelp threads. More delicate flavor than kombu.

WASABI Japanese pale green radish, available as a paste or dried powder (to be mixed with water). Very strong flavor. Used to season sushi and dipping sauces. Sometimes called Japanese mustard.

ZEST The grated outer rind of citrus fruits.

Glossary

amino acid. The result of the body's breakdown of protein, used for body recycling; excess is converted to energy or fat.

angina. Feeling of pressure or pain, mild to severe, in the chest area. Caused by blood-starved heart muscles.

anxiety. Feeling of tension or uneasiness, distress.

aorta. This largest artery (±1" in diameter) funnels blood from the heart (left ventricle) to smaller arteries, which then carry blood to the rest of body.

arterioles. Smallest arteries pass blood to capillaries.

arteriosclerosis. Occurs when artery walls thicken and lose flexibility (see atherosclerosis). Commonly called hardening of the arteries.

atheroma. The collection of fatty plaque in the arteries.

atherosclerosis. A type of arteriosclerosis from fatty plaque deposits on artery walls that block the flow of blood.

atrium (atria). Upper chamber of the heart that receives blood from the body and lungs, passing it to the ventricles.

blood clot. A semisolid, gelatinous mass of coagulated blood that consists of red blood cells, white blood cells and platelets entrapped in a fibrin network. If the clot forms in a blood vessel or in a chamber of the heart it is a thrombus, and the condition is called *thrombosis.*

blood pressure. The measured force on the walls of the arteries as it is pumped from the heart. (See *diastolic, systolic.*)

bradycardia. Too low a heartbeat rate, usually less than 60.

bruit. A murmur caused by a narrowed blood vessel.

capillaries. Smallest branches of blood vessels. Capillaries have thin walls that oxygen and carbon dioxide can pass through.

cardiac arrest. A stopped heartbeat, customarily with loss of consciousness; usually from ventricular fibrillation.

cardiologist/cardiology. Physician/study of the heart and blood vessels, and related disorders and treatments.

cardio-pulmonary resuscitation (CPR). The restoration of blood circulation to prevent death and brain damage, using mouth-to-mouth breathing and heart muscle compression.

cardiovascular. Related to the heart and blood vessels.

catheter. Flexible tube inserted in blood vessels or body duct to deliver medication, drain fluids, diagnose or repair.

cerebral embolism. A stroke caused by a clot traveling to the brain, usually originating elsewhere.

cerebral thrombosis. A stroke caused by a clot in an artery leading to the brain.

cholesterol. A white, fatty matter manufactured by the body; essential for cells, hormone production and other functions; only found in animals and their byproducts. High levels lead to plaque formation and coronary heart disease.

collateral circulation. Occurs when blood vessels join to take over some of the circulation of blocked vessels; natural bypass.

congestive heart failure. Decline of the heart's ability to pump causes fluid accumulation in lungs, stomach and legs.

coronary arteries. Vessels supplying blood to the heart's muscles; name comes from *corona,* Latin for crown.

coronary bypass surgery. Procedure to graft new vessels around blocked arteries to increase flow to heart's muscles.

coronary heart disease. Decreased blood flow to the heart's muscles from narrowing or blockage of coronary arteries.

cyanosis. Poorly oxygenated blood, causing blue skin in lips and fingernails.

diabetes. The inability of the body to process glucose (blood sugar). In Type I, juvenile onset, no insulin is produced. In Type II, adult onset, insulin is not effectively utilized.

diastolic. Relaxing phase of the heartbeat; the second number of blood pressure measurement (systolic/diastolic).

diuretic. Matter that rids the body of excess water and salts.

edema. Swelling of parts of the body due to fluid retention.

electrocardiogram (EKG, ECG). Chart of heart's electrical impulses; used as a diagnostic tool.

embolism (embolus). A clot or particle carried in the bloodstream that blocks the passage of blood.

endocardium. The inner lining of the heart.

fiber. Roughage; type of carbohydrate not broken down in digestion; rarely found in animal products.

fibrin. Protein-based fibers that form clots to block wounds.

glucose. A sugar found in many foods; the body's primary fuel.

heart attack (myocardial infarction). Death of heart muscle resulting from reduction or stoppage of blood flow.

hemoglobin. Substance found in red blood cells; combines with oxygen and carries it to cells.

high density lipoproteins (HDL). Carry cholesterol away from artery walls and help prevent it from depositing there.

hormones. Chemicals that control almost every body function, released into the blood by endocrine glands.

hypercholesterolemia. Very high level of cholesterol.

hyperglycemia. Very high level of glucose (blood sugar).

hypertension. Medical name for high blood pressure.

hypertrophy. Enlarged muscle due to increased work load.

hypoglycemia. Very low level of glucose (blood sugar), most often caused by an overdose of insulin by diabetics.

hypoxia. Lack of sufficient oxygen in body tissue.

inferior vena cava. Major vein in the *lower* body that carries oxygen-depleted blood to the heart.

invasive techniques/procedures. Diagnosis or treatment that enters the body by surgery, catheter or needle puncture.

ischemia. Lack of oxygen in an organ caused by artery blockage.

LDL (low density lipoproteins). Carry cholesterol from the liver to body cells; often called "bad" cholesterol.

lipoproteins. Carry cholesterol and other lipids in the body.

metabolism. Chemical changes and physical processes that allow the body to utilize nutrients needed to sustain life.

monosaturated fats. Fatty acids capable of accepting more hydrogen atoms; remain liquid or soft at room temperature.

multivessel disease. When more than one vein or artery (usually coronary) is impaired or blocked.

myocardial infarction. See **heart attack.**

myocardium. Heart tissue.

noninvasive procedure/technique. Does not require surgery, insertion of a catheter or needle puncture.

open-heart surgery. When the heart's protective sac is opened and a heart-lung machine takes over circulation.

palliative therapy. Treatment to relieve symptoms without attempting to cure the cause.

pericarditis. Inflammation of the heart's protective sac.

pericardium. Heart's outer protective sac (membrane); fluid between this sac and the heart lubricates as it pumps.

phlebitis. Inflammation of veins, usually in the legs.

plaque. Deposits on the inner lining of arteries built up from cholesterol, fats, calcium and other waste in the blood.

platelets. Small cells in the blood. Platelets allow clotting.

polyunsaturated fats. Fatty acids holding the fewest hydrogen atoms; liquid at room temperature.

pulmonary embolism. Blockage of the pulmonary artery or its branches by a clot (embolus).

pulmonary stenosis. Partial or full blockage of the pulmonary artery or valve, usually from plaque.

pulse. Movement of a blood vessel coinciding with the heartbeat.

red blood cells. Cells with hemoglobin that carry oxygen.

renin. Substance that causes blood vessels to contract, regulating blood pressure. Renin is made primarily in the kidneys.

restenosis. Return of blood vessel blockages after treatment.

risk factor. Any behavior or condition (past, present and inherited) increasing the chance of disease or injury.

saturated fats. Fatty acids containing the highest possible number of hydrogen atoms; solid at room temperature.

septum. Strong tissue wall that separates the left and right sides (atria and ventricles) of the heart.

shock. Insufficient blood in vital parts of the body that temporarily stop functioning. If untreated, can lead to brain damage or death; often a reaction to injury.

stasis. Limited or stopped flow.

stenosis. Narrowing of any blood vessel, valve or passage.

stents. Wire scaffold to hold open a tube, such as an artery.

stroke. Stoppage of flow of blood to the brain, usually from a clot or rupture of a blood vessel.

superior vena cava. Major vein in the *upper* body that carries oxygen-depleted blood to the heart.

systolic. Contraction phase of the heartbeat; first number of blood pressure measurement (systolic/diastolic).

tachycardia. Too fast a heartbeat rate, usually greater than 100 beats per minute.

thrombosis. See **blood clot.**

TIA (transient ischemic attack). Very slight stroke, due to a temporary blockage of a blood vessel in the brain. May not be apparent.

triglycerides. Fatty substances (lipids) in the blood and adipose (fatty) tissues; high levels may lead to heart disease.

vasospasm. Sudden involuntary contraction of a blood vessel; abnormal.

vasovagal response. Fainting or light-headedness due to sudden reduction of heartbeat or blood pressure.

vegan. A strict vegetarian who uses no animal products, dairy or eggs. Animal-derived products (leather, silk, etc) also may not be used.

vein. Vessel that returns oxygen-poor blood to the heart.

venous thrombosis. Blood clots in the arteries.

ventricles. Two lower chambers that pump blood to the body (left) and to the lungs (right).

white blood cells (corpuscles). Cells in the blood that destroy harmful bacteria and other foreign substances.

Recommended Resources

Basic Reading

Heidrich, Ruth. *A Race for Life: From Cancer to the Ironman.* Honolulu: Heidrich Weisbrod Associates, 1990.

Kabat-Zinn, Jon, Ph.D. *Full Catastrophe Living: Using the Wisdom of Your Body and Mind to Face Stress, Pain and Illness.* New York: A Delta Book (Dell Publishing), 1990.

McDougall, John A. *McDougall's Medicine, A Challenging Second Opinion.* Piscataway, NJ: New Century Publishers, 1985.

_____. *The McDougall Program, Twelve Days to Dynamic Health.* New York: NAL Books, 1990.

Ornish, Dean. *Dr. Dean Ornish's Program for Reversing Heart Disease.* New York: Ballentine Books, 1991.

Shintani, Terry. *Eat More, Weigh Less Diet.* Honolulu: Halpax Publishing, 1993.

Audio and Video Tapes

Audio tapes are available at or can be ordered from bookstores.

The Art of Meditation by Daniel Goldman (audio)

Jane Fonda's Yoga Exercise Workout (video)

How to Meditate by Lawrence LeShan (audio)

Lilias Yoga for Beginning Students by Lilias Folan (audio/video)

Meditation by Edgar Cayce (audio)

Dr. Dean Ornish's Program for Reversing Heart Disease (audio)

Cookbooks

Recipes in the following are within *Healing Heart* guidelines.

Clark-Grogan, Bryanna. *The "Almost" No-Fat Cookbook.* Summertown, TN: Book Publishing Co., 1994.

Heidrich, Ruth. *The Race for Life Cookbook.* Honolulu: Hawaii Health Publishers, 1994.

McDougall, John and Mary McDougall. *The New McDougall Cookbook.* New York: Dutton, 1993.

Ornish, Dean. *Eat More, Weigh Less.* New York: Harper, 1993.

_____. *Everyday Cooking with Dean Ornish: 150 Seasonal Recipes for Family and Friends.* New York: HarperCollins, 1996.

The following have some recipes that may exceed *Healing Heart* fat recommendations. Most can be modified by leaving out the oil or using a non-fat substitute. Some may may contain animal products. Substitute vegetables for meat and *lite* tofu for dairy.

Bates, Dorothy R. *Tofu Cookbook.* Summertown, TN: Book Publishing Co., 1994.

Crook, William G. and Marjorie Hurt Jones. *Yeast Connection Cookbook —A Guide to Good Nutrition and Better Health.* Jackson, TN: Professional Books/Future Health, 1989.

Metejan, G. *Cooking Without Fat.* Iwindale, CA: Valley Foods, 1992.

Robbins, John. *May All Be Fed.* New York: William Morrow, 1992.

Schlesinger, Sarah. *500 Fat-Free Recipes: A Complete Guide to Reducing the Fat in Your Diet :500 Recipes from Soup to Dessert Containing One Gram of Fat or Less.* New York: Villard Books, 1994.

Shintani, Terry. *Eat More, Weigh Less Cookbook.* Honolulu: Halfax Publishing, 1995.

Shulman, M. *Fast Vegetarian Feasts.* New York: Dial Press, 1981.

_____. *The Vegetarian Feast.* New York: Harper and Row, 1979.

Shurtless, W., and A. Aoyagi, *The Book of Tofu.* Brookline: Autumn Press, 1975.

Southey, P. *The Vegetarian Gourmet Cookbook.* New York: Van Nostrand, 1980.

Stepaniak, Joanne. *The Uncheese Cookbook.* Summertown, TN: Book Publishing Co., 1994.

Information

Patient and Bystander Recognition and Action. National Heart Attack Alert Program, NHLBI, PO Box 30105, Bethesda, MD 20824-0105.

Physicians Committee for Responsible Medicine, PO Box 6322, Washington, DC 20015, (202) 686-2210.

Sports Music, PO Box 769689, Roswell, GA 30076, 800-878-4764.

Vegetarian Resource Group, PO Box 1463, Baltimore, MD 21203, (410) 366-VEGE. Ask for catalog of books, information, helpful items.

Bibliography

Anderson, B.M., R.S. Gibson, J.H. Sabry. "The Iron and Zinc Status of Long-Term Vegetarian Women." *American Journal of Clinical Nutrition,* 1981, 34:1042-1048.

Bailey, C. *The New Fit or Fat.* Boston: Houghton Mifflin, 1991.

_____. *Smart Exercise.* Boston: Houghton Mifflin, 1994.

Barnard, N. *Eat Right, Live Longer.* New York: Harmony Books, 1995.

Bassan, M.M., R.S. Marcus, and W. Ganz. "The Effect of Mild-to-Moderate Mental Stress on Coronary Hemodynamics in Patients with Coronary Artery Disease." *Circulation,* 1980, 65:933-935.

Basset, J.R., K.D. Caincross. "Changes in the Coronary Vascular System Following Prolonged Exposure to Stress." *Pharmacology, Biochemistry and Behavior,* 1977, no 6:311.

Benson, H. "Systemic Hypertension and the Relaxation Response." *New England Journal of Medicine,* 1977, 296:1152 1156.

Benson, H., et al. "Decreased Blood Pressure in Borderline Hypertensive Subjects Who Practiced Meditation." *Journal of Chronic Diseases,* 1974, 27:163-169.

Blacher, R.S., and R.J. Cleveland. "Heart Surgery." *JAMA,* 1979, 242:2463-2464.

Blankenhorn, D.H., and S.H. Brooks. "Angiographic Trials of Lipid-Lowering Therapy." *Arteriosclerosis,* 1981, 1:242-249.

Bourassa, M.G., et al. "Progression of Obstructive Coronary Artery Disease 5 to 7 Years after Aortocoronary Bypass Surgery." *Circulation,* 1778, 58:100-106.

Boyer, J., and F. Kasch. "Exercise Therapy in Hypertensive Men." *JAMA,* 1970, 211:1668-1671.

Brown, M.L., ed. *Present Knowledge in Nutrition.* Washington: International Life Sciences Institute-Nutrition Foundation, 1990.

Burslem, J., et al. "Plasma Apoprotein and Lipoprotein Lipid Levels in Vegetarians." *Metabolism,* 1978, 27:711.

Castelli, W. "HDL-Cholesterol . . . in Coronary Heart Disease." *Circulation,* 1977, 55:767.

Christensen, A., and D. Rankin. *"Easy Does It Yoga."* San Francisco: Harper and Row, 1979.

Committee on Diet and Health. *Diet and Health: Implications for Reducing Chronic Disease Risk.* Washington: National Academy Press, 1989.

Cooper, K. *The Aerobics Program for Total Well-Being.* New York: M. Evans and Co., 1982.

Cooper, M.J. "A Relaxation Technique in the Management of Hypercholesterolemia." *Journal of Human Stress,* 1979, 4:24-27.

Cortis, B. *Heart and Soul, a Psychological and Spiritual Guide to Preventing and Healing Heart Disease.* New York: Villard Books, 1995.

David, M. *Nourishing Wisdom.* New York: Bell Tower Books, 1991.

Dawber, T.R. "Eggs, Serum Cholesterol and Coronary Heart Disease." *American Journal of Clinical Nutrition,* 1982, 36:617.

_____. *The Framingham Study.* Cambridge: Harvard University Press, 1980.

DeBakey, M.E., and A.M. Gotto. *The Living Heart.* New York: Grosset and Dunlap, 1977.

Deutsch, R.M., and M.S. Morrill. *Realities of Nutrition.* Palo Alto: Bull Publishing Company, 1993.

Easwaren, E. *Meditation.* Petaluma, CA: Nilgiri Press, 1978.

Eliot, R.S., and D. Breo. *Is It Worth Dying For? How to Make Stress Work for You, Not against You.* New York: Bantam Books, 1981.

Ellis, F.R., and T. Sanders. "Angina and Vegan Diet" *American Heart Journal,* 1977, 93:805-806.

Enos, W.F., R.H. Holmes, and J. Beyer. "Coronary Disease among United States Soldiers Killed in Action in Korea." Preliminary Report. *JAMA*, 1953, 152:1090.

Flynn, M. "Serum Lipids in Humans Fed Diets Containing Beef or Fish and Poultry." *American Journal of Clinical Nutrition*, 1981, 34:2734.

Food and Nutrition Board, National Research Council. *Recommended Dietary Allowances*. 10th ed. Washington: National Academy Press, 1989.

Frohlich, E.D. "Newer Aspects of Cardiovascular Drugs." *Progressive Cardiovascular Disease*, 1990.

Fuster, V., et al. "Platelet Survival and the Development of Coronary Artery Disease in the Young Adult." *Circulation*, 1981, 63:546.

Goodman, D. "Breaking the Protein Myth." *Whole Life Times*, 1984, July/Aug:26.

Gordon, T. "Diet in Relation to Coronary Heart Disease." *Circulation*, 1981, 63:500.

Gould, K.L. "Changes in Myocardial Perfusion Abnormalities by Position Emission Tomography . . . After Five Years of Risk Factor Modification. JAMA, 1995, 274: 894.

Gould, K.L., et al. "Improved Stenosis Geometry by Quantitative Coronary Arteriography after Vigorous Risk Factor Modification." *American Journal of Cardiology*, 1992, 69(9):845-853.

Haft, J.I., and Y.S. Arkel. "Effect of Emotional Stress on Platelet Aggregation in Humans." *Chest*, 1976, 70:501.

Hallberg, L. "Bioavailability of Dietary Iron in Man." *Annual Review of Nutrition*, 1981, 1:123-147.

Harding, M. "Nutritional Studies of Vegetarians: IV. Fatty Acids and Serum Cholesterol Levels." *American Journal of Clinical Nutrition*, 1962, 10:522.

Harlan, W.R. "Physical and Psychosocial Stress and the Cardiovascular System." *Circulation*, 1981, 63:266A.

Hartley, L.H. "Prescribing Physical Conditioning Activity." *Practical Cardiology*, 1981, 7:119-129.

Heidrich, R.E. *Race for Life: From Cancer to the Ironman*. Kailua, HI: Leslie K. Nunes, 1990.

Helman, A.D., and I. Darnton-Hill. "Vitamin and Iron Status in New Vegetarians." *American Journal of Clinical Nutrition,* 1987, 45:775-778.

Herbert, V. "Separating Food Facts and Myths," in *The Mount Sinai School of Medicine Complete Book of Nutrition.* New York: St. Martin Press, 1990.

Hermann, W. "The Effect of Vitamin E on Lipoprotein Cholesterol Distribution." *Annals of the New York Academy of Sciences,* 1982, 393:467-472.

Jackson, R. "Influence of Polyunsaturated and Saturated Fats." *American Journal of Clinical Nutrition,* 1984, 39:589.

Kabat-Zinn, J. *Full Catastrophe Living: Using the Wisdom of Your Body and Mind to Face Stress, Pain and Illness.* New York: A Delta Book (Dell Publishing), 1990.

Kannel, W. "Serum Cholesterol, Lipoproteins and the Risk of Coronary Heart Disease." *Annals of Internal Medicine,* 1971, 74:1.

Keys, A. "Serum Cholesterol. . .the Effect of Cholesterol in the Diet" *Metabolism,* 1965, 14:776.

_____. *Seven Countries: A Multivariate Analysis of Death and Coronary Heart Disease.* Cambridge: Harvard University Press, 1980.

Kramer, J.R., et al. "Progression of Coronary Atherosclerosis." *Circulation,* 1981, 63:519.

Kritchevsky, D. "Dietary Fiber and other Dietary Factors in Hypercholesteremia." *American Journal of Clinical Nutrition,* 1977, 30:979.

Kurzweil, R. *The 10% Solution.* New York: Crown Publishers, 1993.

Lang, S. "Diet and Disease." *Food Monitor,* 1983, May/June:24.

Latta D., and M. Liebman. "Iron and Zinc Status of Vegetarian and Non-Vegetarian Males." *Nutrition Report International,* 1984, 30:141-149.

Lipid Research Clinic Program. "The Lipid Research Clinics Primary Prevention Trial Results. Reduction in Incidence of Coronary Heart Disease." *JAMA,* 1984, 251:351.

_____. "The Relationship in Reduction of Incidence of Coronary Heart Disease to Cholesterol Lowering." *JAMA,* 1984, 251:365.

Lynch, J.J. *The Broken Heart: The Medical Consequences of Loneliness.* New York: Basic Books, 1977.

Marmot, M.G., et al. "Epidemiological Studies of Coronary Heart Disease and Stroke in Japanese Men Living in Japan, Hawaii and California." *American Journal of Epidemiology*, 1975, 102:514-525.

Martin, B., S. Robinson, and D. Robertshaw. "Influence of Diet on Leg Uptake of Glucose during Heavy Exercise." *American Journal of Clinical Nutrition*, 1978, 31:62-67.

Marx, J.L. "Coronary Artery Spasm and Heart Disease." *Science*, 1980, 208: 1127-1130.

McDougall, J. A. *McDougall's Medicine, A Challenging Second Opinion.* Piscataway, NJ: New Century Publishers, 1985.

_____. *The McDougall Program, Twelve Days to Dynamic Health.* New York: NAL Books, 1990.

McDougall, J. A., and M.A. McDougall. *The McDougall Plan.* Piscataway, NJ: New Century Publishers, 1983.

McGee, D., and T. Gordon. "The Results of the Framingham Study Applied to Four Other U.S.-Based Epidemiologic Studies of Coronary Heart Disease." *The Framingham Study*, Section 31. DHEW Pub. No. (NIH) 76-1083. Washington: National Institutes of Health, 1976.

McNamara, J.J., et al. "Coronary Artery Disease in Combat Casualties in Vietnam." *JAMA*, 1971, 216:1185.

Miettenin, M. "Effect of Cholesterol-Lowering Diet on Mortality from Coronary Heart Disease." *Lancet*, 1972, 2:835.

National Academy of Sciences. *Diet, Nutrition and Cancer.* Washington: National Academy Press, 1982.

O'Brien, B. "Human Plasma Lipid Responses to Red Meat, Poultry, Fish and Eggs." *American Journal of Clinical Nutrition*, 1980, 33:2573.

Ornish, D. "Can Life-Style Changes Reverse Coronary Atherosclerosis?" *Hospital Practice*, 991, 26(5): 123-126, 129-132.

_____. "Can Lifestyle Changes Reverse Coronary Heart Disease?" *World Review of Nutrition & Dietetics*, 1993, 72:38-48.

_____. "Mind/Heart Interactions: For Better and for Worse." *Health Values*, 1978, 2:266-269.

_____. "Reversing Heart Disease through Diet, Exercise, and Stress Management: An Interview with Dean Ornish." *Journal of the American Dietetic Association*, 1991, 91(2):162-165.

_____. "What if Americans Ate Less Fat?" *JAMA*, 1992, 267:362-364.

Ornish D., et al. "Can Lifestyle Changes Reverse Coronary Heart Disease? The Lifestyle Heart Trial." *Lancet*, 1990, 336(8708):129-133.

_____. "Lifestyle Changes and Heart Disease." *Lancet*, 1990, 336(8717):741-742.

Ornish, D., et al. "Effects of Stress Management Techniques and Dietary Changes in Treating Ischemic Heart Disease." *Clinical Research*, 1979, 49:1008.

Ornish, D., et al. "Effects of a Vegetarian Diet and Selected Yoga Techniques in the Treatment of Coronary Heart Disease." *Clinical Research*, 1979, 27:720A.

Paffenbarger, R.S., and W.E. Hale. "Work Activity and Coronary Heart Mortality." *New England Journal of Medicine*, 1975, 292:545.

_____. "Yoga and Biofeedback in the Management of Stress in Hypertensive Patients." *Clinical Science and Molecular Medicine*, 1975, 171s-174s.

Patel, C.H. "Reduction of Serum Cholesterol and Blood Pressure in Hypertensive Patients by Behavior Modification." *Journal of the Royal College of General Practitioners*, 1976, 26:211-215.

Pitchford, Paul. *Healing with Modern Foods, Oriental Traditions and Modern Nutrition.* Berkeley: North Atlantic Books, 1993.

Reader's Digest. *Family Guide to Natural Medicine.* Pleasantville, NY: Reader's Digest Association,1993.

Ribeiro, J. "The Effectiveness of a Low Lipid Diet . . . Coronary Artery Disease." *American Heart Journal*, 1984, 108:1183.

Reisin, E., et al. "Effect of Weight Loss without Salt Restriction on the Reduction in Blood Pressure in Overweight Hypertensive Patients." *New England Journal of Medicine*, 1978, 198:1-6.

Robbins, John. *Diet for a New America.* Walpole, NH: Stillpoint Publishing, 1987.

_____. *May All Be Fed.* New York: William Morrow, 1992.

Ross, R., and J.A. Glomset "The Pathogenesis of Atherosclerosis." *New England Journal of Medicine*, 1976, 295: 369-377, 420-425.

Roth, D., and W.J. Kosstuk. "Noninvasive and Invasive Demonstration of Spontaneous Regression of Coronary Artery Disease Following Aortocoronary Saphenous Vein Bypass Surgery." *American Journal of Cardiology,* 1975, 58:166-170.

Sachs, F.M., W.P. Castelli, and E.H. Kass. "Blood Pressure in Vegetarians." *New England Journal of Medicine,* 1974, 100:390-398.

Sachs, F.M., et al. "Effect of Ingestion of Meat on Plasma Cholesterol of Vegetarians." *JAMA,* 1981, 246:640.

Satchinanda, S. *Integral Hatha Yoga.* New York: Holt, Rinehart and Winston, 1970.

Schekelle, R.B., et al. "Diet, Serum Cholesterol, and Death from Coronary Heart Disease: The Western Electric Study." *New England Journal of Medicine,* 1981, 304:65-70.

Schiffer, F., et al. "Evidence for Emotionally-Induced Coronary Arterial Spasm in Patients with Angina Pectoris." *British Heart Journal,* 1980, 44:62-66.

Sirtori, C.R., et al. "Clinical Experience with the Soybean Protein Diet in the Treatment of Hypercholesterolemia." *American Journal of Clinical Nutrition,* 1979, 32:1645-1667.

Small, D.M. "Cellular Mechanisms for Lipid Deposition in Atherosclerosis." *New England Journal of Medicine,* 1977, 297:873.

Stamler, J. "Lifestyles, Major Risk Factors, Proof and Public Policy." *Circulation,* 1978, 58:3-19.

Taik Lee, K. "Geographical Studies of Atherosclerosis: The Effects of a Strict Vegan Diet." *Archives of Environmental Health,* 1962, 4:14.

Thomas, G.S., et al. *Exercise and Health: the Evidence and the Implications.* Cambridge: Oelgeschlager, Gunn and Hain, Inc., 1981.

Verani, M.S., et al. "Effects of Exercise Training on Left Ventricular Performance and Myocardial Perfusion in Patients with Coronary Artery Disease." *American Journal of Cardiology,* 1981, 47:797-803.

Weil, A. *Spontaneous Healing.* New York: Knopf/Random House, 1995.

Zaret, B.L., et al., eds. *Yale University School of Medicine Heart Book.* New York: Hearst Books, 1992.

Index of Recipes

Index

About the Author

D r. Neal Pinckney is a graduate of the University of Southern California and of Oxford University, where he received his Ph.D. in clinical and educational psychology. He has done post-doctoral work at Stanford and Vienna Universities and has taught at the University of California, Davis; the University of Hawaii; and the California State University, Sacramento, where he was chairman of the Department of Behavioral Sciences and retired as emeritus professor. He maintained a private practice in family and individual therapy and psychoanalysis for almost 30 years, and was psychologist to the California Highway Patrol for 13 years. He now lives in rural Hawaii.

Following a diagnosis of severe heart blockage, his doctors strongly recommended bypass surgery. Through lifestyle changes, he reversed his condition without surgery.

Dr. Pinckney is the founder and director of the Healing Heart Foundation, which offers free support groups that provide education on how to reverse and prevent heart disease without surgery. He walks over four miles and bicycles over 12 miles a day, and practices yoga and meditation. His cholesterol level has dropped more than 240 points, and his blood pressure is normal.

Dr. Pinckney is the author of *A Casebook of Law and Ethics in Counseling and Psychotherapy* (California State

University Press, 1986) and is a contributor and an editor of the four-volume *Encyclopedia of Psychology, Second Edition* (John Wiley & Sons, 1994).

Dr. Pinckney would be pleased to hear from persons interested in reversing heart disease through lifestyle changes and through support groups that help people accomplish this goal. Letters may be addressed to the Healing Heart Foundation, 84-683 Upena Street, Makaha, HI 96792, and e-mail sent to heart@aloha.net.